Standardized Training In Swallowing Physiology — Evidence-Based Assessment Using The Modified Barium Swallow Impairment Profile (MBSImP™) Approach

Bonnie Martin-Harris, Ph.D., CCC-SLP, BCS-S, ASHA Fellow

Professor, Department of Otolaryngology-Head and Neck Surgery, College of Medicine
Professor, Department of Health Science and Rehabilitation, College of Health Professions
Director, Ph.D. Program in Health and Rehabilitation Science, College of Health Professions
Director, MUSC Evelyn Trammell Institute for Voice and Swallowing
Medical University of South Carolina, Charleston, SC

Northern Speech Services
Gaylord, Michigan

Standardized Training in Swallowing Physiology — Evidence-Based Assessment Using the Modified Barium Swallow Impairment Profile (MBSImP™) Approach

© 2015 Northern Speech Services. All rights reserved.

Published by Northern Speech Services, Inc., P. O. Box 1247, Gaylord, MI 49735.

All rights reserved, including the right to reproduce this book or portions thereof in any form or by any means, electronic or mechanical, including photocopying, recording, or by any information storage and retrieval system, without the permission in writing from the publisher. All inquiries should be addressed to Northern Speech Services, Inc., P. O. Box 1247, Gaylord, MI 49735.

The Modified Barium Swallow Impairment Profile (MBSImP™) protocol and online training are property of the Medical University of South Carolina (MUSC) and under exclusive management by Northern Speech Services, Inc (NSS). © 2008 & © 2011 Medical University of South Carolina. All rights reserved.

Printed in the United States of America.

ISBN 978-1-935578-31-4

Acknowledgments

The author wishes to acknowledge the following individuals for their invaluable contributions:

Kendrea L. Focht, Ph.D., C.Sc.D., CCC-SLP, Department of Otolaryngology-Head and Neck Surgery, Medical University of South Carolina, Charleston, SC, for her research and development of tables, manual organization, and detailed editing.

William G. Pearson, Jr., Ph.D., Clinical Anatomist, Assistant Professor, Department of Cellular Biology and Anatomy, Medical College of Georgia, Georgia Regents University, Augusta, GA, for his expert anatomical knowledge of the upper aerodigestive tract.

Emma Vought, M.S., Medical Illustrator and Animator, Clinical Instructor, Department of Neurosciences, College of Medicine, Medical University of South Carolina, Charleston, SC, for her high quality medical illustrations.

Kate Humphries, M.S., CCC-SLP, Department of Otolaryngology-Head and Neck Surgery Medical University of South Carolina, Charleston, SC, for her assistance in collecting fluoroscopic and animation images.

Marty Brodsky, Ph.D., Sc.M., CCC-SLP, Assistant Professor, Department of Physical Medicine and Rehabilitation, Johns Hopkins University School of Medicine for his assistance in collecting fluoroscopic and animation images.

David H. McFarland, Ph.D., Professor, School of Speech-Language Pathology and Audiology, Faculty of Medicine, Université de Montréal, Adjunct Professor, School of Communication Sciences and Disorders, Faculty of Medicine, McGill University, for his contributions to the conceptualization of the content.

Thomas Slominski, Sr., M.A., CCC-SLP, Thomas Slominski, Jr., John Sandidge, M.A., CCC-SLP, and the rest of the team at Northern Speech Services, Gaylord, MI, for their help, advice and support in the preparation and publication of this work.

Medical University of South Carolina, Department of Otolaryngology–Head and Neck Surgery and Evelyn Trammell Institute for Voice and Swallowing for the support and privilege to care for patients who drive our clinical research: Dr. Paul Lambert, Chair, Drs. Terry Day, Boyd Gillespie, Josh Hornig, Eric Lentsch, and Judy Skoner from our head and neck surgical team, Drs. Lucinda Halstead and Ashli O'Rourke, Heather Bonilha, Ph.D., CCC-SLP, and Julie Blair, M.A., CCC-SLP, BCS-S from our laryngology team, our speech-language pathologists, and Anita Cheslek who keeps us organized and grounded in patient centered care.

TABLE OF CONTENTS

Acknowledgments 1
Abbreviations 4
INTRODUCTION 5
    MBSImP Physiologic Components of Swallowing Impairment 6
    Purpose of the MBSS and MBSImP Approach 7
    Why Standardization? 8
    A Note about Aspiration 12

FUNCTIONAL DOMAINS OF SWALLOWING IMPAIRMENTS

Introduction to Components of Swallowing Impairment 13
    Oral Domain 15
        Component 1 – Lip Closure 15
        Component 2 – Tongue Control during Bolus Hold 17
        Component 3 – Bolus Preparation/Mastication 20
        Component 4 – Bolus Transport/Lingual Motion 24
        Component 5 – Oral Residue 27
        Component 6 – Initiation of Pharyngeal Swallow 32
    Pharyngeal Domain 35
        Component 7 – Soft Palate Elevation 35
        Component 8 – Laryngeal Elevation 37
        Component 9 – Anterior Hyoid Excursion 42
        Component 10 – Epiglottic Movement 45
        Component 11 – Laryngeal Vestibular Closure 48
        Component 12 – Pharyngeal Stripping Wave 52
        Component 13 – Pharyngeal Contraction 55
        Component 14 – Pharyngoesophageal Segment Opening 58
        Component 15 – Tongue Base Retraction 61
        Component 16 – Pharyngeal Residue 64
    Esophageal Domain 67
        Component 17 – Esophageal Clearance 67
References 71

Abbreviations

2-D	two-dimensional
3-D	three-dimensional
A/P	anterior-posterior
C1	cervical spinal nerve 1
CN	cranial nerve
V	trigeminal nerve
V_2	maxillary branch of CN V
V_3	mandibular branch of CN V
VII	facial nerve
IX	glossopharyngeal nerve
X	vagus nerve
XII	hypoglossal nerve
CPM	cricopharyngeus muscle
LES	lower esophageal segment
MBSImP	Modified Barium Swallow Impairment Profile
MBSS	modified barium swallow study
OI	overall impression
PAS	Penetration-Aspiration Scale
PES	pharyngoesophageal segment
PESO	pharyngoesophageal segment opening
SLP	speech-language pathologist

INTRODUCTION

The **Modified Barium Swallow Impairment Profile (MBSImP™)**[1] is a standardized approach to instruction, assessment, and reporting of physiologic swallowing impairment based on observations from videofluoroscopic images obtained during a modified barium swallow study (MBSS). The MBSImP was developed and tested during a five-year supported study by the National Institutes of Health and requires standardized *training*, standardized *administration protocol*, standardized *interpretation and scoring*, and standardized *reporting*. The details of the study are described in our 2008 publication in Dysphagia, which is available online at http://www.ncbi.nlm.nih.gov/pmc/articles/PMC4217120/.

Swallowing is a complex physiologic function that requires interactions between and within body systems. Therefore, the assessment of functional swallowing requires consideration and quantification of multiple physiologic, patient, social, and environmental factors. This learning resource will focus on the *physiologic factors* requisite for the execution of normal swallowing. These **physiologic factors** have been and continue to be tested for their association with other important factors such as general health, diet, nutrition, and quality of life.

The physiologic components (items) of swallowing impairment included in the MBSImP were derived from evidence available in a large body of literature and through expert consensus. The components were grouped into functional domains based on their strong, yet non-redundant relationships with one another found during statistical testing. There are 17 components distributed across three functional domains of swallowing, with each component on the MBSImP contributing uniquely to judgments of overall swallowing impairment.

---

[1] B. Martin-Harris B, Brodsky MB, Michel Y, et al. MBS measurement tool for swallow impairment – MBSImp: establishing a standard. Dysphagia. 2008;23(4):392-405.

NOTE: References that contributed to this manual are provided at the conclusion of the manual and are not embedded within the text.

MBSImP Physiologic Components of Swallowing Impairment

Oral Domain
1. Lip closure
2. Tongue control during bolus hold
3. Bolus preparation/mastication
4. Bolus transport/lingual motion
5. Oral residue
6. Initiation of pharyngeal swallow

Pharyngeal Domain
7. Soft palate elevation
8. Laryngeal elevation
9. Anterior hyoid excursion
10. Epiglottic movement
11. Laryngeal vestibular closure
12. Pharyngeal stripping wave
13. Pharyngeal contraction
14. Pharyngoesophageal segment opening
15. Tongue base retraction
16. Pharyngeal residue

Esophageal Domain
17. Esophageal clearance in upright position

The Oral Domain includes components that relate to oral containment, motion of the oral tongue, and oral clearance. The Pharyngeal Domain includes components relating to pharyngeal bolus clearance and airway protection. Lastly, the Esophageal Domain includes only one component that falls within the speech language pathologist's (SLP's) scope of practice – esophageal bolus clearance in the upright position. This component is included because of the known association between impaired esophageal clearance and oropharyngeal swallowing behavior.

Purpose of the MBSS and MBSImP Approach

The purpose of the MBSS (rapid, dynamic fluoroscopic imaging of the upper aerodigestive tract in the upright or semi-upright position) and MBSImP approach is to:

- identify and distinguish the type and severity of physiologic swallowing impairment(s),

- provide surrogate information (sensation, weakness, pressure, etc.) regarding the sensorimotor mechanisms that underpin swallowing impairment,

- determine the presence, cause, and response to airway invasion (penetration/aspiration),

- and assess the compensations and adaptations of structural movements and bolus flow to evidence-based interventions.

The MBSS is *not a feeding assessment*. The goal of any radiologic imaging that introduces X-ray exposure to patients should be to maximize diagnostic and clinical yield while minimizing radiation exposure. Varied consistencies are tested in a selective way, because evidence supports the existence of modifications in oropharyngeal and esophageal physiology and airway protection using standardized contrast (barium) consistencies. Barium consistencies administered during the MBSS *do not* match exactly all of the potentially multiple and varied consistencies that may be included in a patient's meal. Rather, inherent in the MBSImP approach is the ability for the *like-trained* clinician to make reliable judgments about swallowing physiology based on a standardized set of barium consistencies shown to influence oropharyngeal swallowing function. From this information, the trained clinician is able to judge how the swallowing mechanism will function with food choices, such as mixed textures, meat, and breads, without having to introduce each material during the MBSS. Not only are there safety issues related to infection control, prolonged radiation exposure, and adverse consequences of aspiration when using these materials during the MBSS, they are not necessary to formulate clinical impressions about physiologic impairment or oral intake decisions. For example, if a patient scores a (3) on Component 6 (i.e., initiation of the pharyngeal swallow at the level of the pyriform sinus) and scores a (3) on Component 2 (i.e., more than half of the bolus escapes posteriorly during attempted bolus containment), clearly the patient will have difficulty with foods that are characterized by a mixture of liquids, solids, or semisolids. Further, clinical decisions regarding oral intake require integrated knowledge not only of swallowing physiology, but also cognitive-communication status, availability of necessary supervision, and other environmental and social factors. Intake and diet consistency decisions may be guided by the MBSImP physiologic metrics but *will not be prescribed* from the scores because of the varied factors contributing to safe and functional oral intake. The MBSS is a window in time and requires follow-up observations of the patient during mealtime or therapeutic feeding sessions when appropriate.

Why Standardization?

It is generally accepted that standardized practices in health care facilitate patient safety, continuity of care, and clinical outcome data that are unambiguous and measurable. Standardized training and practices improve clinician confidence and performance, better protect liability of the provider, improve compliance with practice and reporting, and contain cost. Like any area of assessment in health care, standardization of the MBSS protocol does not prevent judicious individual variation to facilitate personalized care plans. However, wide variations in practice result in examination recommendations that may be unsafe, cannot be compared or assessed for their validity, or cannot be objectively modified for performance and process improvement. Accuracy and patient safety are dependent on standardized training, accuracy and reliability of physiologic judgments, appropriate acquisition and recording instrumentation, use of standardized contrast materials, and standardized reporting – all of which are necessary to capture and communicate the complex physiologic and bolus flow movements that occur during normal and impaired swallowing.

Swallowing assessment should be conducted by like-trained clinicians with similar specialty training and credentials from programs with standardized curriculums that include rigorous competency assessment. There is clearly a role for interprofessional education and practice in the management of dysphagic patients; however, the physiologic assessment falls in the purview of specialists trained in the function of the upper aerodigestive tract and communication-cognitive processes that are intimately involved in safe and efficient eating and drinking. Critical decisions about swallowing function, impairment, and eating and drinking can be life changing and life threatening. Hence, training in the implementation and interpretation of the MBSS should be standardized to optimize patient outcomes, and clinicians should be accountable for demonstration of accurate physiologic assessment and treatment planning. The fluoroscopic equipment must be capable of continuous fluoroscopy or 30 pulses per second. Current data show that fluoroscopy settings and recording rates influence the details necessary for accurate assessment of swallowing physiology that subsequently influence treatment decisions.

The MBSImP protocol has been standardized and tested, and thus, should be administered for each patient whenever possible. We have demonstrated that adherence to the protocol improves the efficiency of the exam without increasing radiation exposure time. There will be instances, however, when some viscosities or volumes are not deemed safe for administration based on the patient's clinical status or performance on a preceding swallow. Average fluoroscopy exposure time for clinicians trained in the MBSImP approach is 2.89 minutes, which includes the introduction of compensatory strategies. Multiple trials have not proven necessary to capture impressions of impairment for the 17 MBSImP components. We have also demonstrated that a trained clinician is able to capture impairment by observing components across bolus consistencies/swallow trials to formulate overall impression (OI) scores for each swallowing component. The OI score was designed to capture impairment even when all trials are not possible during the MBSS.

In addition to standardization of training in swallowing physiology and interpretation of assessment findings, every attempt should be made to standardize the radiographic data acquisition, recording, and viewing methods (lateral and anterior-posterior (A/P) views). Despite attempts for optimal patient positioning during the MBSS, not all structures may be visualized as planned because of physical or cognitive constraints of the patient. However, the clinician should exercise diligence to take reasonable steps to capture the physiologic swallowing continuum from lips through esophagus. The optimal lateral view includes the lips anteriorly, the nasal cavity superiorly, the posterior pharyngeal wall posteriorly, and the cervical esophagus and upper tracheal air column inferiorly.

Oropharyngeal physiology is dependent on the nature of the task, the instructions given, and bolus volume and viscosity. Therefore, when considering the physiology of swallowing, the implementation of a standardized approach will result in accurate observations of the targeted component. Presentation order, manner, instruction, and volume of the standardized barium preparations used in the MBSImP protocol are presented on page 11.

Clinicians understandably ask how a protocol can be standardized in the presence of patients who are so functionally diverse. The scoring system has a built-in method to account for boluses not given because of swallowing severity or physician order. Swallows that employ compensatory strategies or swallowing maneuvers are scored separately and not included in the baseline OI scores; however, the potential change in the scoring metric provides immediate evidence for improvement in physiology and clinical yield from the MBSS.

MBSImP validated protocol (presentation order, manner, volume, and instruction).

Viewing Plane	Trial Number	Bolus Viscosity	Bolus Volume	Clinician Instruction
Lateral	1	Thin Liquid	5-mL (tsp.)	"Hold this in your mouth until I ask you to swallow." Once bolus hold is achieved, participant instructed to "Swallow."
	2		5-mL (tsp.)	"Hold this in your mouth until I ask you to swallow." Once bolus hold is achieved, participant instructed to "Swallow."
	3		Single cup sip	"Take a sip as you normally would, but hold it in your mouth until I ask you to swallow." Once bolus hold is achieved, participant instructed to "Swallow."
	4		Sequential swallow	"Drink this in your usual manner until I tell you to stop."
	5	Nectar-Thick Liquid	5-mL (tsp.)	"Hold this in your mouth until I ask you to swallow." Once bolus hold is achieved, participant instructed to "Swallow."
	6		Single cup sip	"Take a sip as you normally would, but hold it in your mouth until I ask you to swallow." Once bolus hold is achieved, participant instructed to "Swallow."
	7		Sequential swallow	"Drink this in your usual manner until I tell you to stop."
	8	Honey-Thick Liquid	5-mL (tsp.)	"Hold this in your mouth until I ask you to swallow." Once bolus hold is achieved, participant instructed to "Swallow."
	9	Pudding	5-mL (tsp.)	"Swallow."
	10	Cookie	½ cookie coated with 3-mL pudding	"Chew this as you normally would and swallow."
Anterior-Posterior	11	Nectar-Thick Liquid	5-mL (tsp.)	"Hold this in your mouth until I ask you to swallow." Once bolus hold is achieved, participant instructed to "Swallow."
	12	Pudding	5-mL (tsp.)	"Swallow."

A Note about Aspiration

The MBSS is not a *"pass or fail test"* based on the presence or absence of aspiration. Inappropriate reference to these terms undermines the critical purposes and value of the examination. Aspiration is justifiably a primary concern or risk factor when evaluating the ability of a patient to safely and efficiently eat and drink. Aspiration is the entry of food, liquid, saliva, sputum, refluxate, or other ingested material into the airway. These substances should rarely approach the laryngeal vestibule and never routinely pass through the vocal folds in healthy, awake individuals. Patients with reduced pulmonary defense mechanisms (e.g., cough, mucociliary clearance, etc.) are at risk for acquiring pulmonary infection such as aspiration pneumonia – a disease with high morbidity and leading cause of death in the elderly. Despite the grave consequences associated with aspiration pneumonia in dysphagic patients, data would support that the majority of patients seen in a teaching or community-based hospital do not present with pneumonia at the time of the MBSS. This is likely because the role of swallowing clinicians is early detection of swallowing impairment and prevention of aspiration pneumonia through comprehensive assessments followed by an appropriately guided management plan. The benefits are well recognized by the health care community and patients are referred earlier in the course of their disease or condition. Aspiration is *neither a necessary or sufficient* measure of swallowing impairment, because swallowing impairment can exist without accompanying aspiration observed during a MBSS. Our work has repeatedly demonstrated that if aspiration detection serves as the sole goal of the MBSS, we would miss approximately 2/3 of patients who have physiologic swallowing impairments that could potentially improve using targeted, evidence-based interventions. Detection of aspiration is a radiographic sign of ingested material in the airway. The goal is to determine the underlying physiologic cause of aspiration, which then serves as the focus of targeted intervention or restoration.

Scores for airway invasion are not included in the MBSImP scoring metrics, and it is recommended that the validated Penetration-Aspiration Scale (PAS) be used in conjunction with the MBSImP to capture this important, but different information regarding swallowing safety.

FUNCTIONAL DOMAINS OF SWALLOWING IMPAIRMENTS

Introduction to Components of Swallowing Impairment

Swallowing is a synergistic motor response to multiple sensory inputs applied to the regions of the oropharyngeal cavities and esophageal body. The oropharyngeal swallowing system is physiologically linked to the respiratory system and behaviorally manifests as respiratory cessation (pause) or inhibition typically during the expiratory phase of the breathing cycle. Temporal synchronization of respiratory flow, kinematic, and videofluoroscopic signals have demonstrated that optimal patterns and timing exists for respiratory cessation, airway closure, and pharyngeal clearance during swallowing. Normal swallows occur most frequently during cessation in the expiratory phase of the breathing cycle between middle and low expiratory lung volumes, with some variability related to characteristics of the ingested material and nature of the swallowing task.

Swallowing is primarily a positive pressure phenomenon, with pressures generated by multiple muscles and structures applied to the tail of the bolus throughout the upper aerodigestive tract. The bolus is contained in the oral cavity (if appropriate), and pressures are applied to the bolus tail by the oral tongue, in addition to composite pressures produced by apposition of the tongue base, soft palate, and anteriorly and laterally displaced pharyngeal walls (i.e., shortening and stripping). The efficiency for bolus pressure generation will be decreased whenever there is loss of pressure in either the oral or pharyngeal cavities, such as in the case of incomplete lip closure, incomplete soft palate elevation and retraction, incomplete pharyngeal contraction, or an open supraglottis at the height of the swallow (i.e., the point of maximal muscle contraction and structural displacement). Loss of pressure will result in the bolus taking a path of least resistance through the anterior oral cavity, nasopharynx, upper airway, or paretic (weakened) side of a pharynx. These swallowing inefficiencies will be exacerbated when there is downstream resistance to bolus flow; for instance, in the case of decreased distention and/or duration of the pharyngoesophageal segment (PES) related to impaired biomechanics of the larynx and pharynx, or intrinsic structural anomalies (e.g., cricopharyngeal disorders, radiation fibrosis, scarring). As the clinician views the videofluoroscopic image, there must be a keen awareness of the structures that apply these normal pressures in order to accurately determine bolus viscosity/

volume, postural, and other eating/drinking strategies that compensate for or facilitate improvement in oropharyngeal pressures. Further, the mechanisms of pressure loss should be directly targeted using strengthening, endurance, and range-of-motion training or sensory-based interventions during swallowing treatment or surgical restoration that follow the MBSS.

Reduction in swallowing pressures, muscle weakness, and sensory loss cannot be directly assessed from a MBSS. Evidence from studies that directly measured sensation and pressure simultaneously with videofluoroscopic recording, however, support the clinical practice of using MBSS observations (surrogates) to indirectly assess the integrity of pressure, strength, and sensation. From these observations, a targeted treatment plan can be developed. Decisions regarding the need for direct measurements of pressure (e.g., manometry) or observations of structures (e.g., endoscopy, sensory testing) can be made based on the results of the MBSS.

Oral Domain
Component 1 – Lip Closure

Lip closure is a critical element of oral bolus containment, and thereby important for the function, pleasure, and aesthetics associated with eating and drinking. The sealed lips not only prevent escape of the bolus from the anterior oral cavity, but also contribute to a closed oral cavity allowing for the generation of intra-oral pressures that lead to efficient bolus transport.

The muscle(s) implicated as primary contributor(s) to the function of each component is/are bolded in the tables throughout the manual.

Table 1 Muscles associated with MBSImP Component 1 – Lip Closure

Functional Group	Name	Innervation	Action
Lips	**Orbicularis oris**	CN VII	Lip seal Anterior oral containment
	Levator labii superioris		
	Levator labii superior alaeque nasi		
	Levator anguli oris		
	Zygomaticus minor		
	Zygomaticus major		
	Risorius		
	Depressor anguli oris		
	Depressor labii inferioris		
	Mentalis		

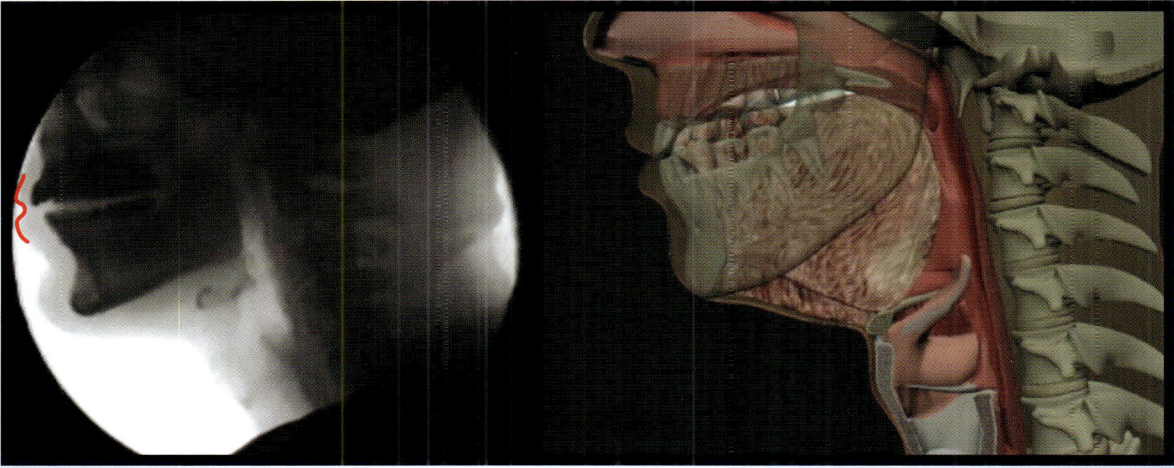

Figure 1 Videofluoroscopic and 3-D animated images demonstrating Component 1 – Lip Closure.

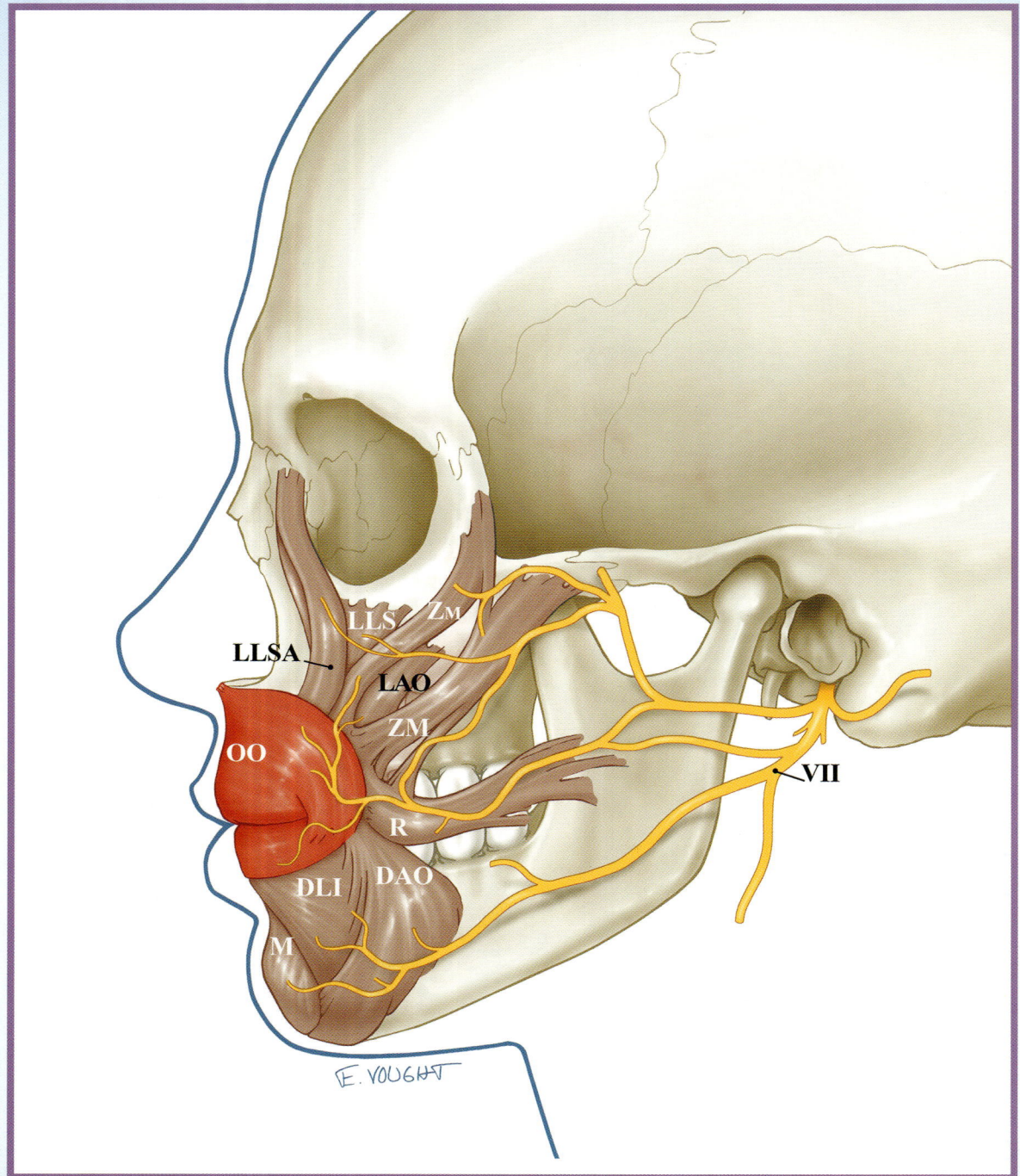

Figure 2 Muscles and innervation of Component 1 – Lip Closure. DAO-Depressor anguli oris; DLI-Depressor labii inferioris; LAO-Levator anguli oris; LLSA-Levator labii superior alaeque nasi; LLS-Levator labii superioris; M-Mentalis; OO-Orbicularis oris; R-Risorius; ZM-Zygomaticus major; Zm-Zygomaticus minor. VII refers to the facial nerve.

Oral Domain
Component 2 – Tongue Control during Bolus Hold

A healthy, non-dysphagic adult has the capability to control and contain a liquid bolus within the oral cavity, which is accomplished by complete elevation and approximation of the anterior, lateral, and posterior margins of the tongue (back of oral tongue) to the hard and inferiorly-anteriorly displaced soft palate. Sensation to the tongue and palate also contribute to oral bolus containment. Although this containment may not be characteristic of all liquid swallows, including larger volumes during sequential drinking, years of clinical experience and testing have shown that the ability to contain a bolus in the oral cavity is a positive prognostic indictor for effective application of various swallowing treatments. For example, if a patient cannot contain a bolus within the oral cavity (due to a sensorimotor/structural tongue or cognitive impairment) and the clinician provides instruction to tuck the chin because of a delay in pharyngeal swallow initiation, the material will fall deep in the pharynx and misdirect to the airway during the swallow. Given this role in swallowing safety, the integrity of the tongue-to-palatal seal should be tested with a simple verbal command. During administration of liquid boluses (thin, nectar-thickened, and honey-thickened liquids) using the M3SImP protocol, the patient is cued to "hold this in your mouth until I ask you to swallow." The integrity of tongue control during bolus hold is observed prior to initiation of any productive tongue movement to propel the bolus through the oral cavity.

Table 2 Muscles associated with MBSImP Component 2 – Tongue Control during Bolus Hold

Functional Group	Name	Innervation	Action
Intrinsic muscles of the tongue	Superior longitudinal	CN XII	Shapes the tongue to hold and control bolus
	Inferior longitudinal		
	Transverse		
	Vertical		
Soft palate muscle	Tensor veli palatini	CN V	Stiffens the soft palate Facilitates posterior oral containment
Extrinsic muscles of the tongue	Palatoglossus	CN X	Closes entry to oropharynx via raising the back of the tongue and drawing down the palate to form the glossopalatal seal Facilitates posterior oral containment
	Genioglossus	CN XII	Shapes the tongue to hold and control bolus
Suprahyoid muscles	Geniohyoid	C1	Stabilizes the floor of mouth
	Mylohyoid	CN V	

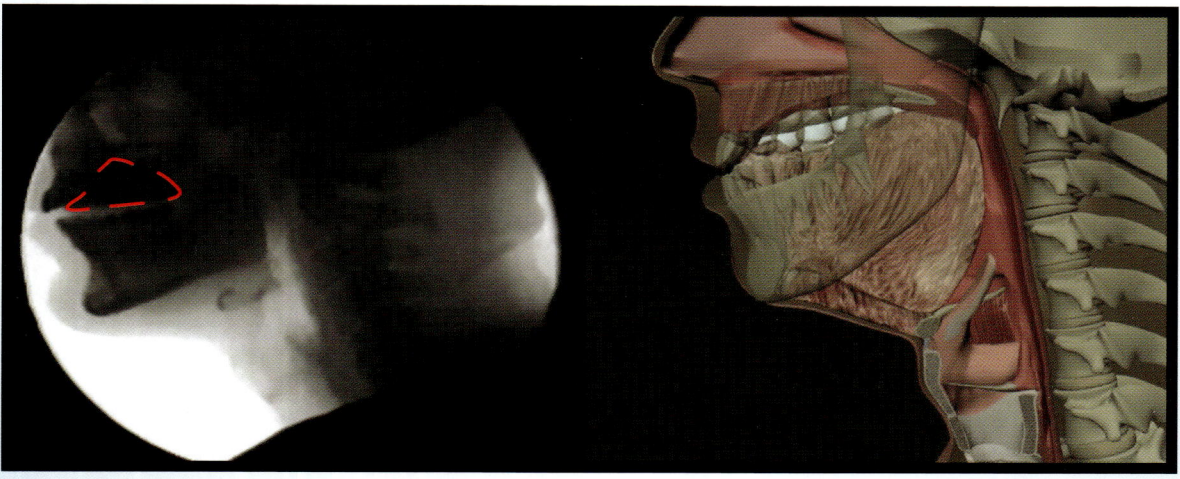

Figure 3 Videofluoroscopic and 3-D animated images demonstrating Component 2 – Tongue Control during Bolus Hold.

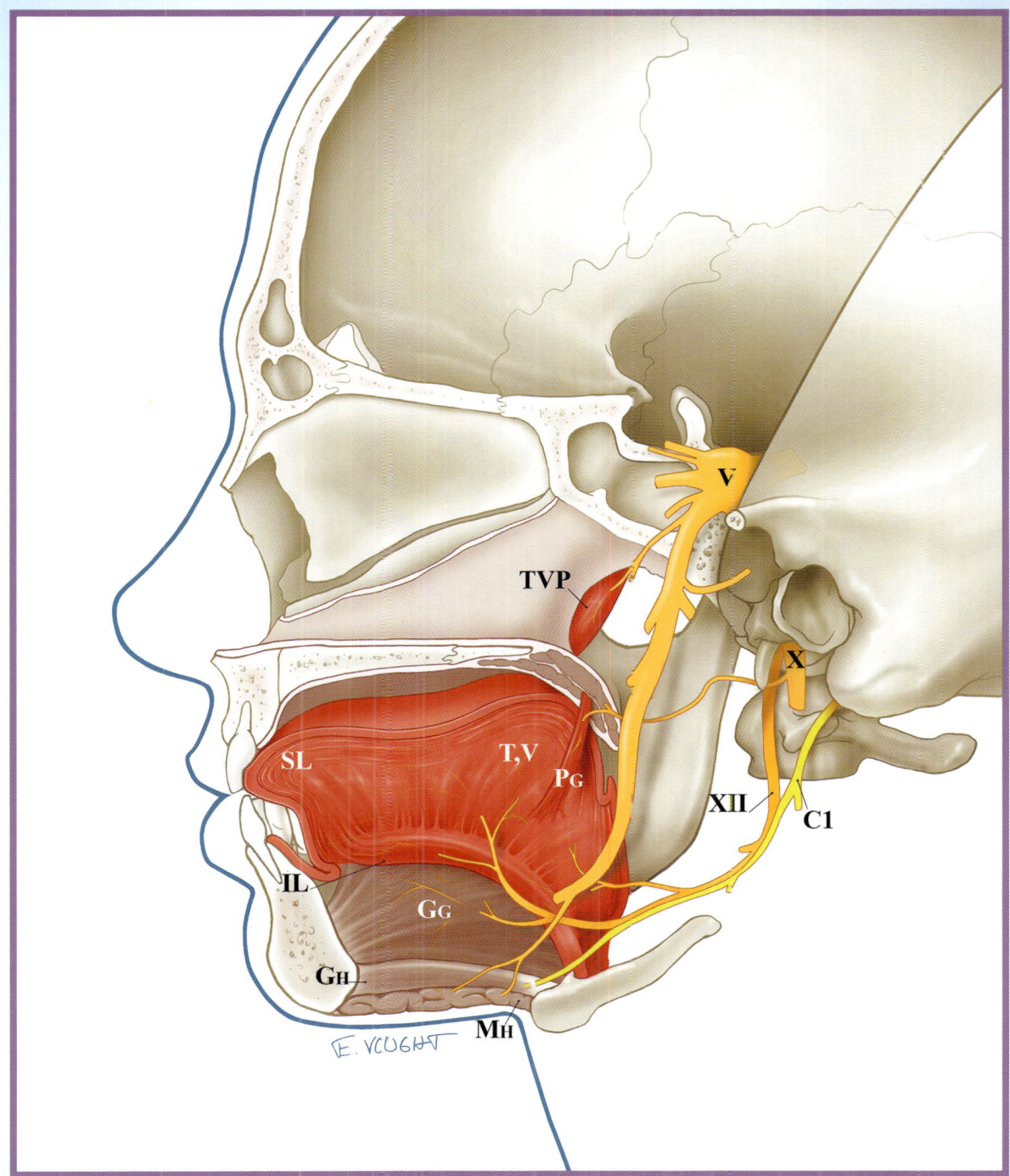

Figure 4 Muscles and innervation of Component 2 – Tongue Control during Bolus Hold.
GG-Genioglossus; GH-Geniohyoid; IL-Inferior longitudinal (tongue); MH-Mylohyoid; PG-Palatoglossus; SL-Superior longitudinal (tongue); T,V-Transverse, Vertical (tongue); TVP-Tensor veli palatini. V, X, and XII refer to trigeminal, vagus, and hypoglossal nerves, respectively. C1 refers to cervical spinal nerve 1.

Oral Domain
Component 3 – Bolus Preparation/Mastication

Preparation and mastication of a semisolid or solid bolus provides the greatest pleasure involved during eating as an individual acutely tastes and smells the foods being ingested. The bolus is mixed with saliva and manipulated in the oral cavity to the margins of the teeth for mastication (chewing). Rotary chewing motions of the jaw serve to break down the bolus into pieces that will be efficiently and safely propelled through the pharynx and esophagus. Further, coordinated tongue movements are highly integrated into the masticatory process.

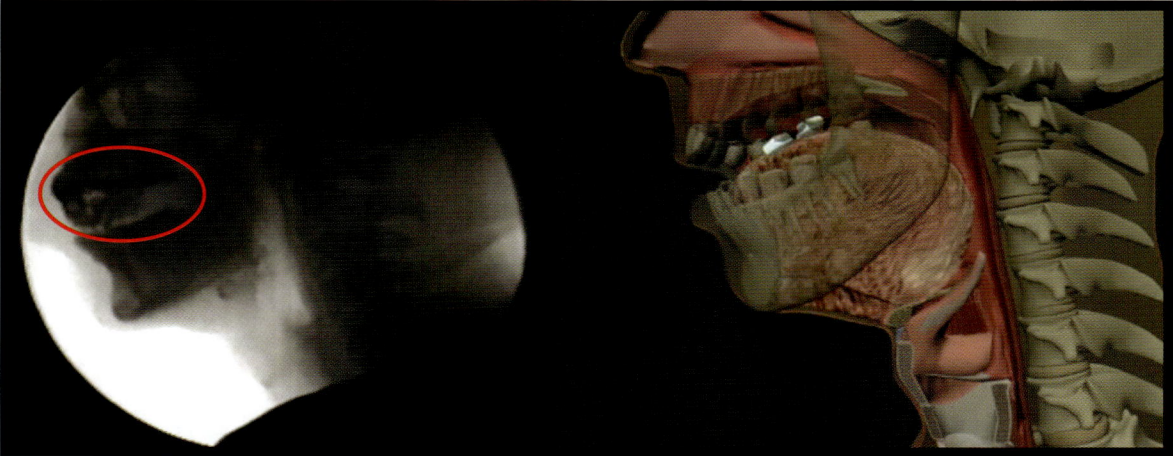

Figure 5 Videofluoroscopic and 3-D animated images demonstrating Component 3 – Bolus Preparation/Mastication.

Table 3 Muscles associated with MBSImP Component 3 – Bolus Preparation/Mastication

Functional Group	Name	Innervation	Action
Muscles of mastication	Masseter	CN V	Elevates the mandible to close the mouth
	Pterygoids		Medial: Elevates the mandible to close the mouth
			Lateral: Side-to-side (rotary) movement of the mandible
	Temporalis		Elevates the mandible to close the mouth
Intrinsic muscles of the tongue	Superior longitudinal	CN XII	Moves the bolus to surface of the teeth for chewing and assists in bolus formation
	Inferior longitudinal		
	Transverse		
	Vertical		
Extrinsic muscles of the tongue	Genioglossus	CN XII	Moves the tongue laterally
	Hyoglossus		Depresses the tongue
	Styloglossus		Posterior oral containment
	Palatoglossus	CN X	
Facial muscle	Buccinator	CN VII	Compresses the cheeks against the teeth
Suprahyoid muscles	Geniohyoid	C1	Stabilizes the floor of mouth to assist with chewing efficiency and tongue movement
	Mylohyoid	CN V	Depresses the mandible to open the mouth
	Digastricus	Anterior belly: CN V Posterior belly: CN VII	Stabilizes the floor of mouth to assist with chewing efficiency and tongue movement
	Stylohyoid	CN VII	Stabilizes the floor of mouth to assist with chewing efficiency and tongue movement
Muscles of the lips	Orbicularis oris	CN VII	Lip seal Anterior oral containment
	Levator labii superioris		
	Levator labii superior alaeque nasi		
	Levator anguli oris		
	Zygomaticus minor		
	Zygomaticus major		
	Risorius		
	Depressor anguli oris		
	Depressor labii inferioris		
	Mentalis		

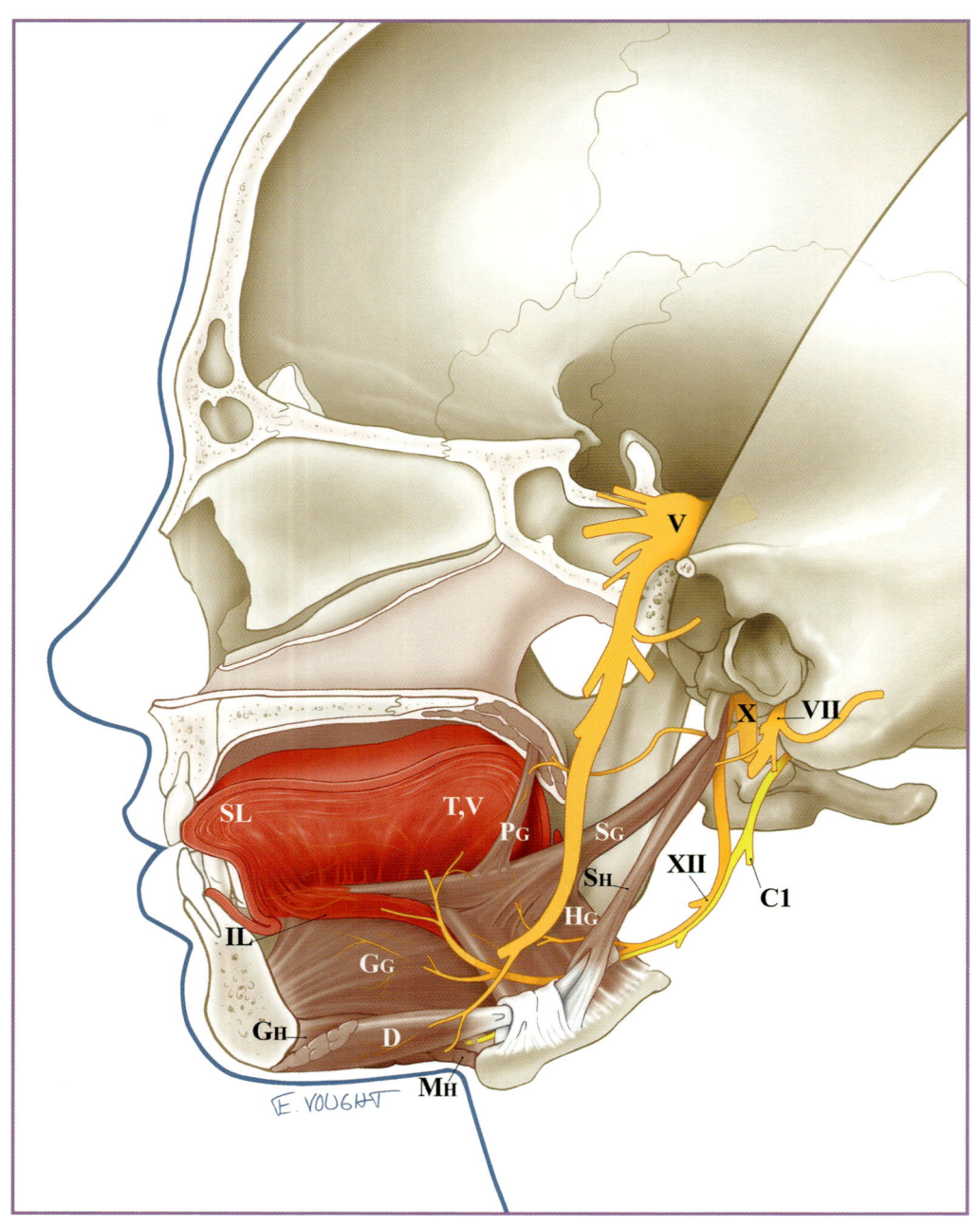

Figure 6 Muscles and innervation of Component 3 – Bolus Preparation/Mastication.
B-Buccinator; D-Digastricus (anterior belly); DAO-Depressor anguli oris; DLI-Depressor labii inferioris; GG-Genioglossus; GH-Geniohyoid; HG-Hyoglossus*; IL-Inferior longitudinal (tongue); LAO-Levator anguli oris; LLSA-Levator labii superior alaeque nasi; LLS-Levator labii superioris; MA-Masseter; M-Mentalis; MH-Mylohyoid; OO-Orbicularis oris; P-Pterygoids; PG-Palatoglossus*;

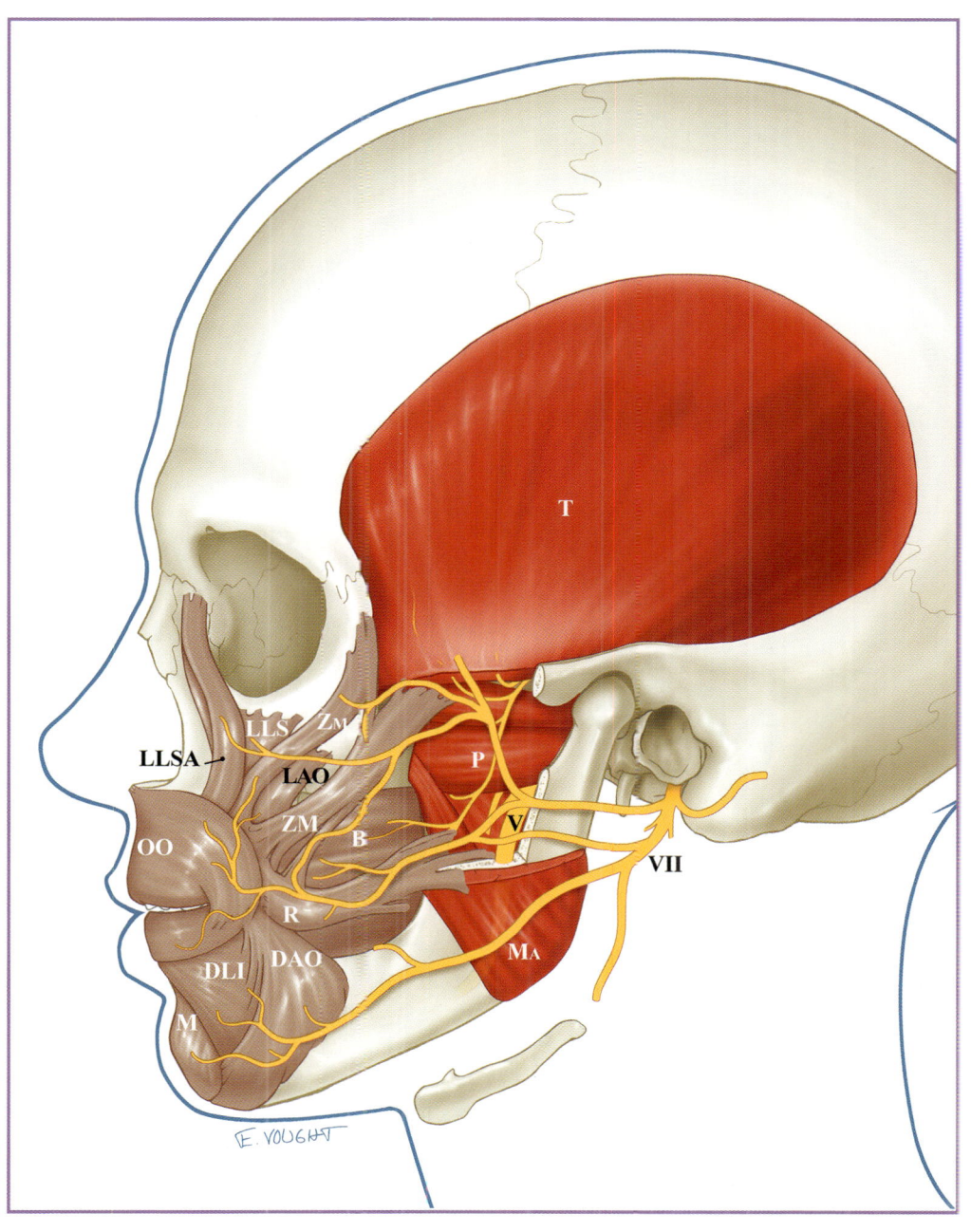

R-Risorius; SG-Styloglossus*; SH-Stylohyoid; SL-Superior longitudinal (tongue); T-Temporalis; T,V-Transverse, Vertical (tongue) ZM-Zygomaticus major; ZM-Zygomaticus minor. V, VII, X, and XII refer to trigeminal, facial, vagus, and hypoglossal nerves, respectively. C1 refers to cervical spinal nerve 1. *Muscle is superimposed on a paramidsagittal cut-away of the tongue. NOTE: The posterior belly of digastricus muscle is not pictured.

Oral Domain
Component 4 – Bolus Transport/Lingual Motion

Bolus transport through the oral cavity is characterized by progressive, anterior-posterior elevation and approximation of the tongue body to the palate that applies pressure to the bolus tail. This motion is brisk, coordinated without delay, and results in clearance of the oral cavity and bolus passage to the oropharynx.

Table 4 Muscles associated with MBSImP Component 4 – Bolus Transport/Lingual Motion			
Functional Group	**Name**	**Innervation**	**Action**
Intrinsic muscles of the tongue	**Superior longitudinal**	CN XII	Presses the tongue against the palate to move the bolus posteriorly. Maintains cohesive shape of bolus between the tongue and palate
	Inferior longitudinal		
	Transverse		
	Vertical		
Extrinsic muscles of the tongue	Genioglossus	CN XII	Positions the tongue against the palate to move the bolus posteriorly
	Hyoglossus		
	Styloglossus		
	Palatoglossus	CN X	
Suprahyoid muscles	Geniohyoid	C1	Stabilizes the floor of mouth to maximize efficiency of tongue movement
	Mylohyoid	CN V	
	Digastricus	Anterior belly: CN V	
	Stylohyoid	CN VII	

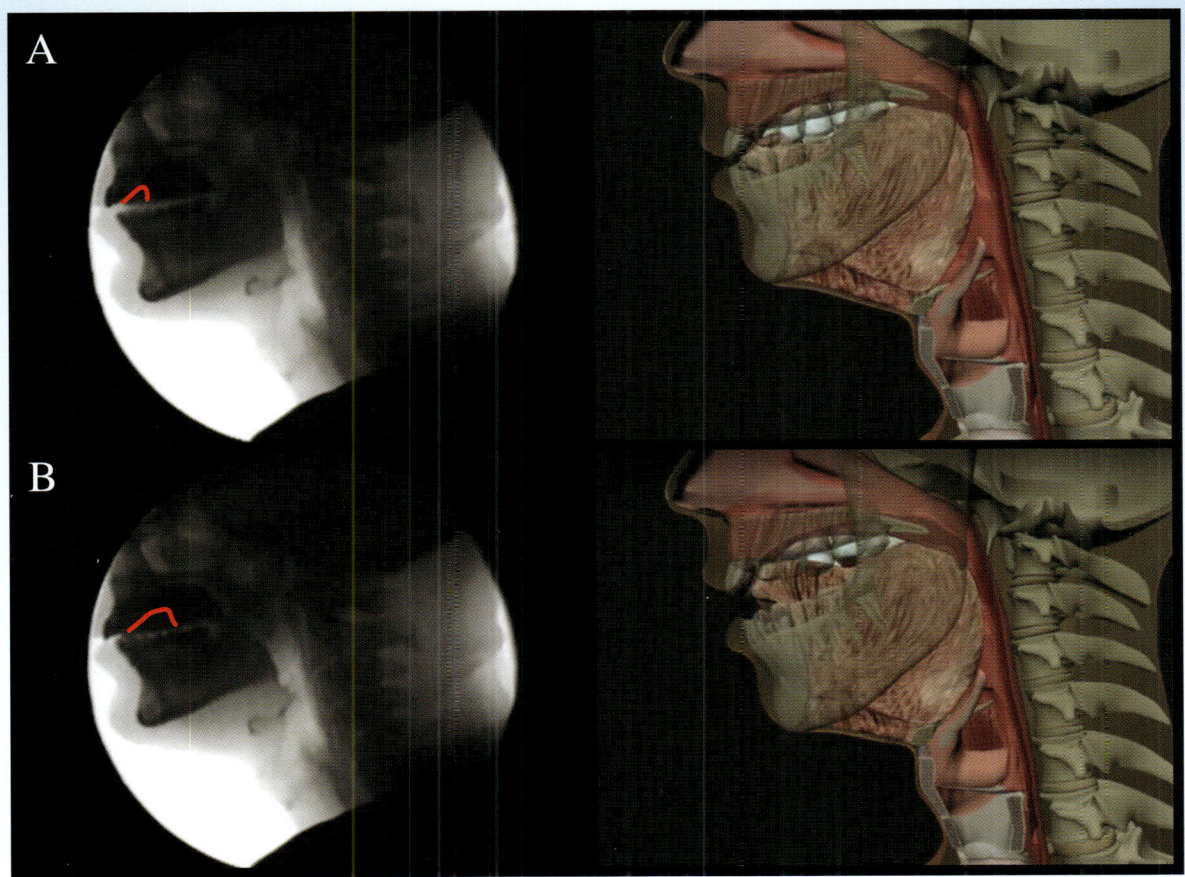

Figure 7 Videofluoroscopic and 3-D animated images demonstrating Component 4 – Bolus Transport/Lingual Motion. (A) Initiation of bolus transport. (B) Transport of bolus posteriorly towards oropharynx.

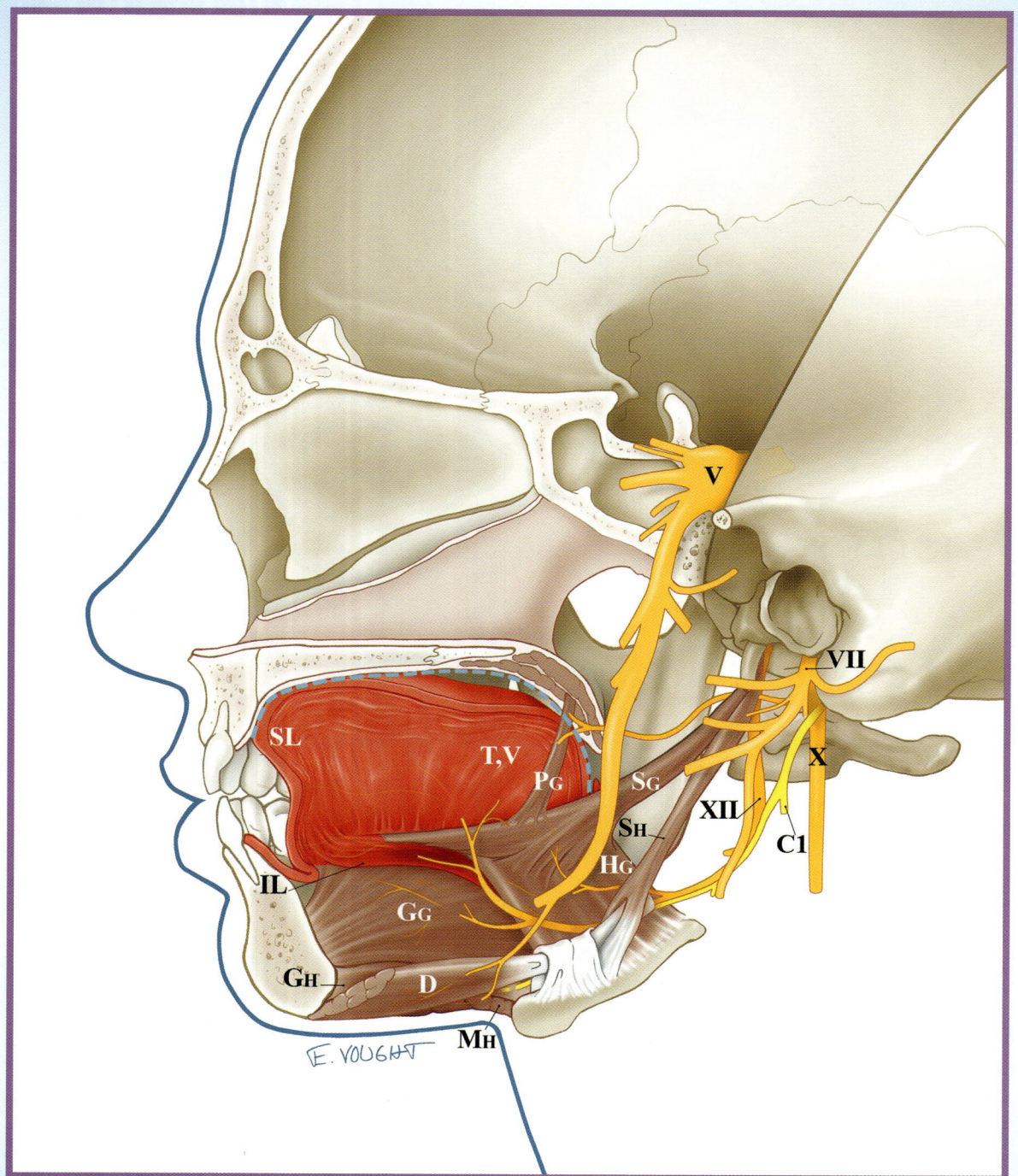

Figure 8 Muscles and innervation of Component 4 – Bolus Transport/Lingual Motion. D-Digastricus (anterior belly); GG-Genioglossus; GH-Geniohyoid; HG-Hyoglossus; IL-Inferior longitudinal (tongue); MH-Mylohyoid; PG-Palatoglossus; SG-Styloglossus; SH-Stylohyoid; SL-Superior longitudinal (tongue); T,V-Transverse, Vertical (tongue). V, VII, X, and XII refer to trigeminal, facial, vagus, and hypoglossal nerves, respectively. C1 refers to cervical spinal nerve 1.

Oral Domain
Component 5 – Oral Residue

Unlike the majority (15 of 17) of components of impairment observed on the MBSImP, oral residue is not a physiologic action. Rather, residue represents a radiographic sign of a physiologic impairment that our studies have demonstrated is significantly associated with other impaired components in the oral domain and several patient outcome measures. Despite the limitations of attempting to make three-dimensional (3-D) cavity observations from a two-dimensional (2-D) view, we were able to develop a metric that demonstrated good reliability and external validity. Oral residue represents any contrast beyond coating of the oral structures remaining in the oral cavity following swallow completion. Multiple sensorimotor features of the tongue and orofacial region contribute, but intact lingual motion (Component 4) is the primary element of oral clearance.

Table 5 Muscles associated with MBSImP Component 5 – Oral Residue

Functional Group	Name	Innervation	Action
Intrinsic muscles of the tongue	**Superior longitudinal**	CN XII	Collects and shapes the bolus, and then transports bolus posteriorly
	Inferior longitudinal		
	Transverse		
	Vertical		
Muscles of mastication	Pterygoids	CN V	Stabilizes the floor of mouth to maximize efficiency of tongue movement
	Masseter		
	Temporalis		
	Buccinator	CN VII	Compresses the cheeks against the teeth
Extrinsic muscles of the tongue	Genioglossus	CN XII	Positions the tongue against the palate to move the bolus posteriorly
	Hyoglossus		
	Styloglossus		
	Palatoglossus	CN X	
Suprahyoid muscles	Geniohyoid	C1	Stabilizes the floor of mouth to maximize efficiency of tongue movement
	Mylohyoid	CN V	
	Digastricus	Anterior belly: CN V	
	Stylohyoid	CN VII	

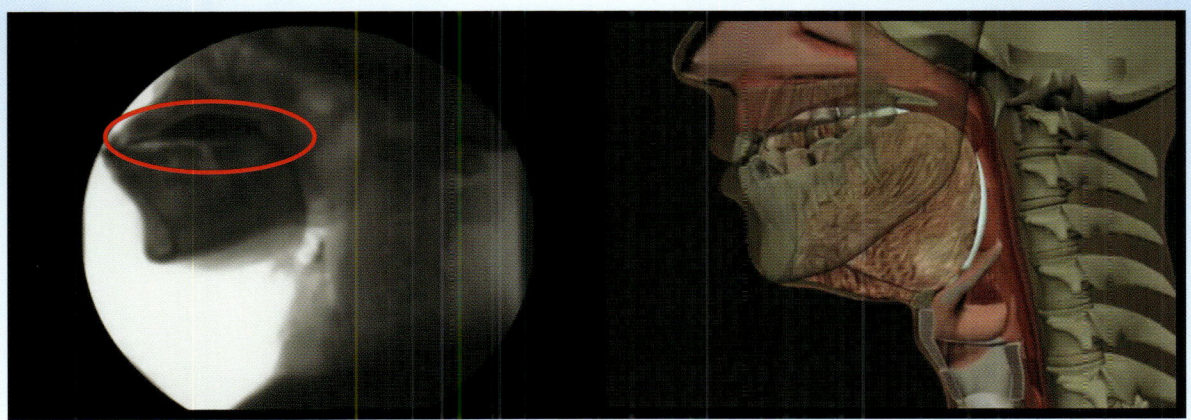

Figure 9 Videofluoroscopic and 3-D animated images demonstrating Component 5 – Oral Residue.

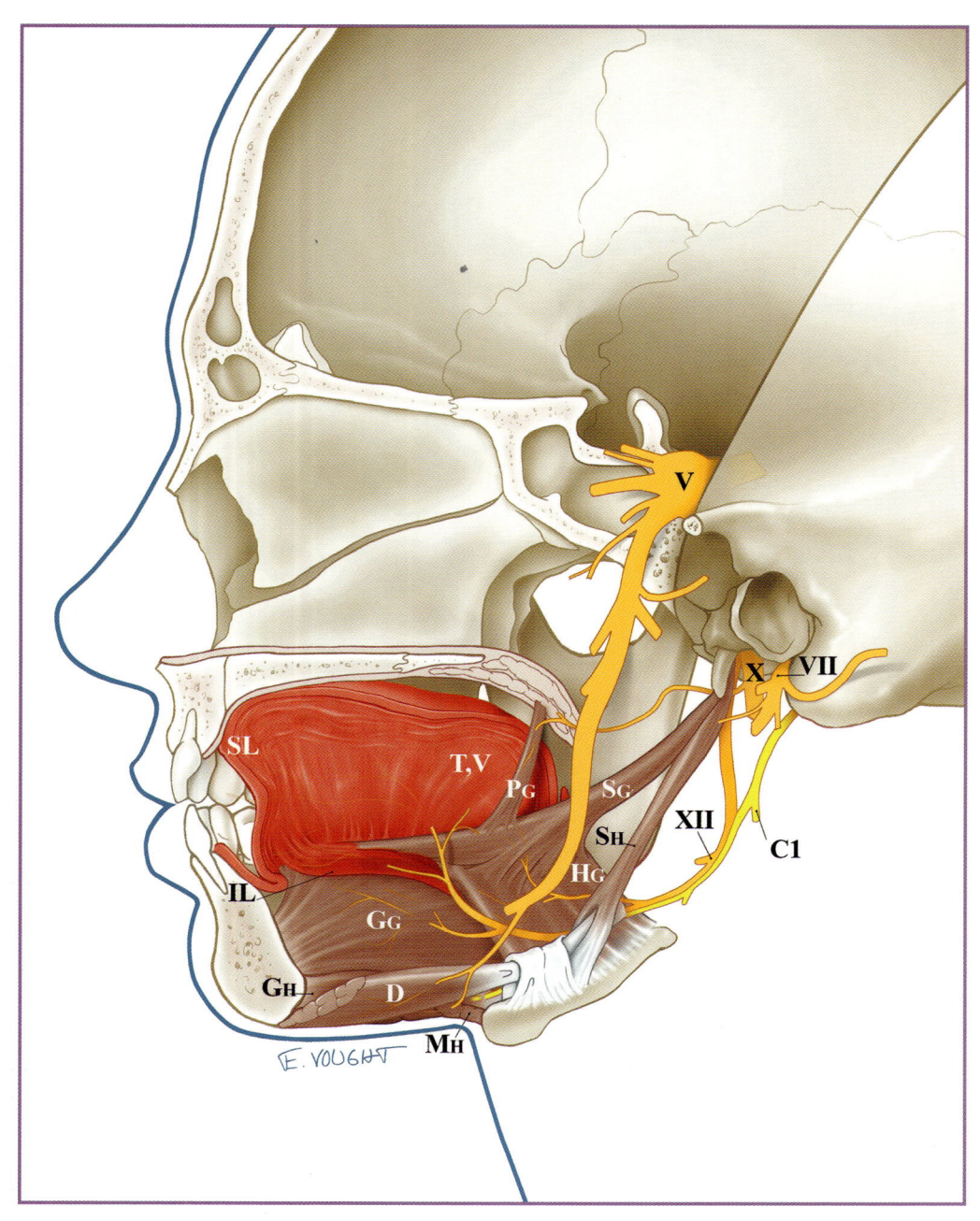

Figure 10 Muscles and innervation of Component 5 – Oral Residue. B-Buccinator; D-Digastricus (anterior belly); GG-Genioglossus; GH-Geniohyoid; HG-Hyoglossus; IL-Inferior longitudinal (tongue); M-Masseter; MH-Mylohyoid; P-Pterygoids; PG-Palatoglossus; SG-

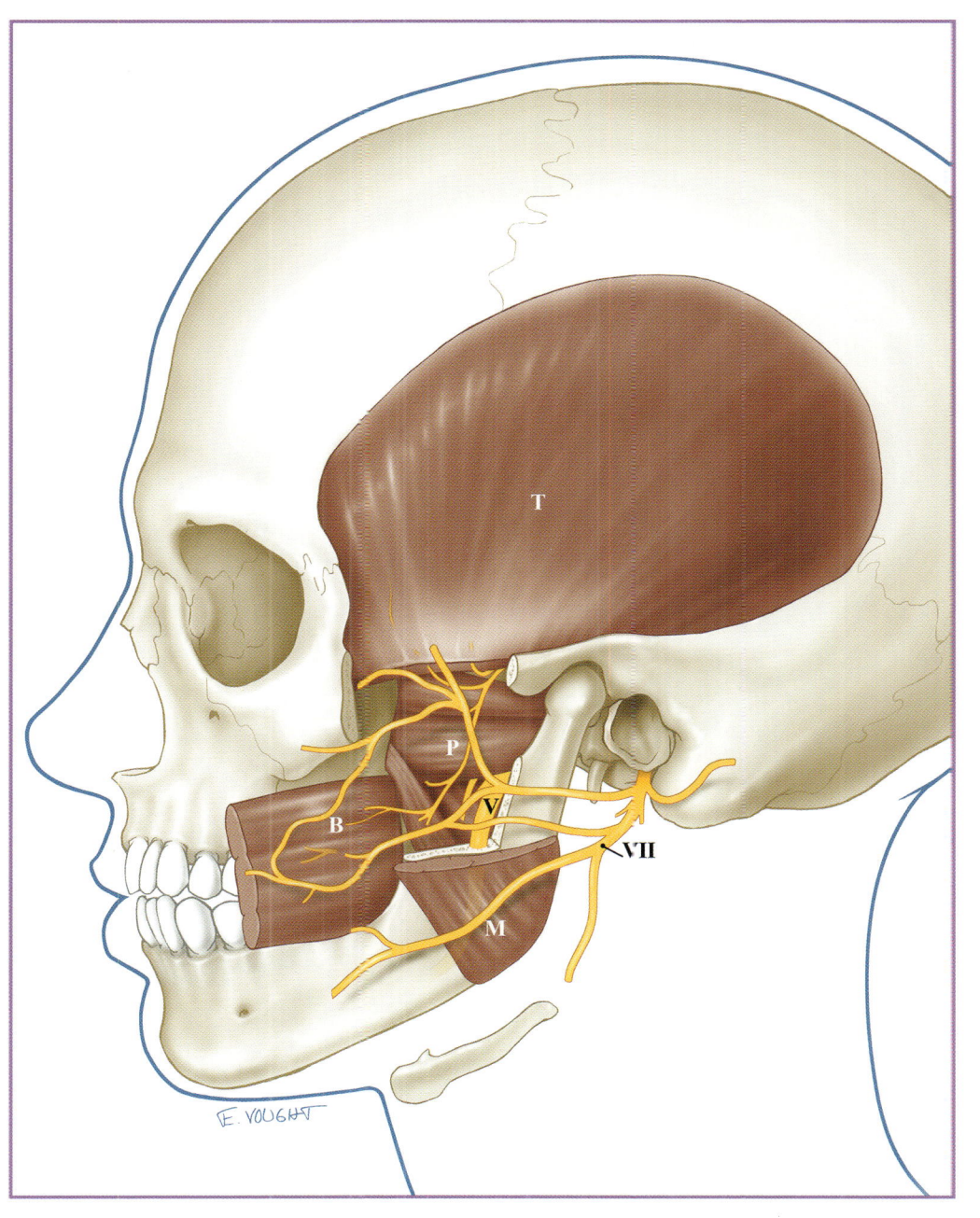

Styloglossus; SH-Stylohyoid; SL-Superior longitudinal (tongue); T-Temporalis; T,V-Transverse, Vertical (tongue). V, VII, X, and XII refer to trigeminal, facial, vagus, and hypoglossal nerves, respectively. C1 refers to cervical spinal nerve 1.

Oral Domain
Component 6 – Initiation of Pharyngeal Swallow

The onset of the initiation of the pharyngeal swallow is signaled on the MBSS by the first brisk movement of the superior-anterior hyoid trajectory and has been described as a motor response to a multiplicity of sensory inputs, including pressures associated with movement of the tongue, presence of a bolus, and to a lesser degree, taste and temperature. The motor response includes soft palatal elevation and retraction (Component 7), laryngeal elevation (Component 8), (superior) anterior hyoid movement (Component 9), epiglottic inversion (Component 10), laryngeal vestibular closure (Component 11), pharyngeal stripping wave (Component 12), pharyngeal contraction (Component 13), pharyngoesophageal segment opening (PESO) (Component 14), and tongue base retraction (Component 15). The initiation of hyoid trajectory should be rapid and uninterrupted. Because initiation of the pharyngeal swallow is a response to sensory inputs, the sensory receptive fields in the oropharynx are primarily implicated as the mechanisms that receive afferent information supplied by the tongue and bolus and subsequently carry this information to the (bilateral) swallowing centers in the medulla. Activity of the commanding sensorimotor nuclei in the brainstem is modulated by cortical structures that effect the execution of the pharyngeal swallow.

Table 6 Cranial nerves innervating sensory receptive fields associated with MBSImP Component 6 – Initiation of Pharyngeal Swallow

Sensory Receptive Fields	Innervation	Branch	Action
Glossopharyngeal (faucial) arches Back of tongue	CN IX	Pharyngeal branch	Initiation of pharyngeal swallow
Base of tongue Valleculae Epiglottis Pharyngeal wall Aryepiglottic folds Ventricular folds Arytenoids True vocal folds Pyriform sinuses	CN X	Superior laryngeal nerve, internal branch	

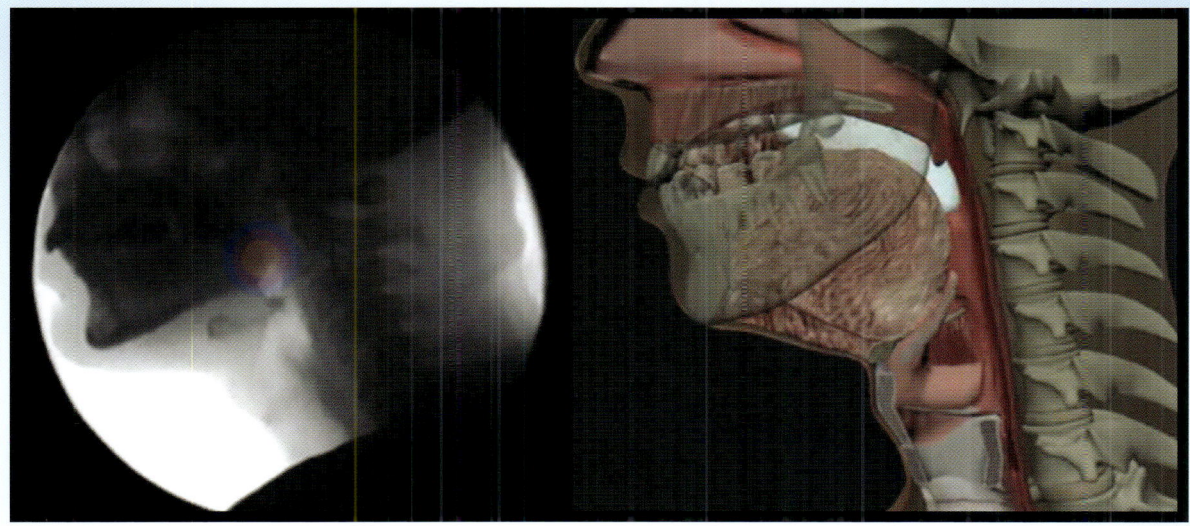

Figure 11 Videofluoroscopic and 3-D animated images demonstrating Component 6 – Initiation of Pharyngeal Swallow.

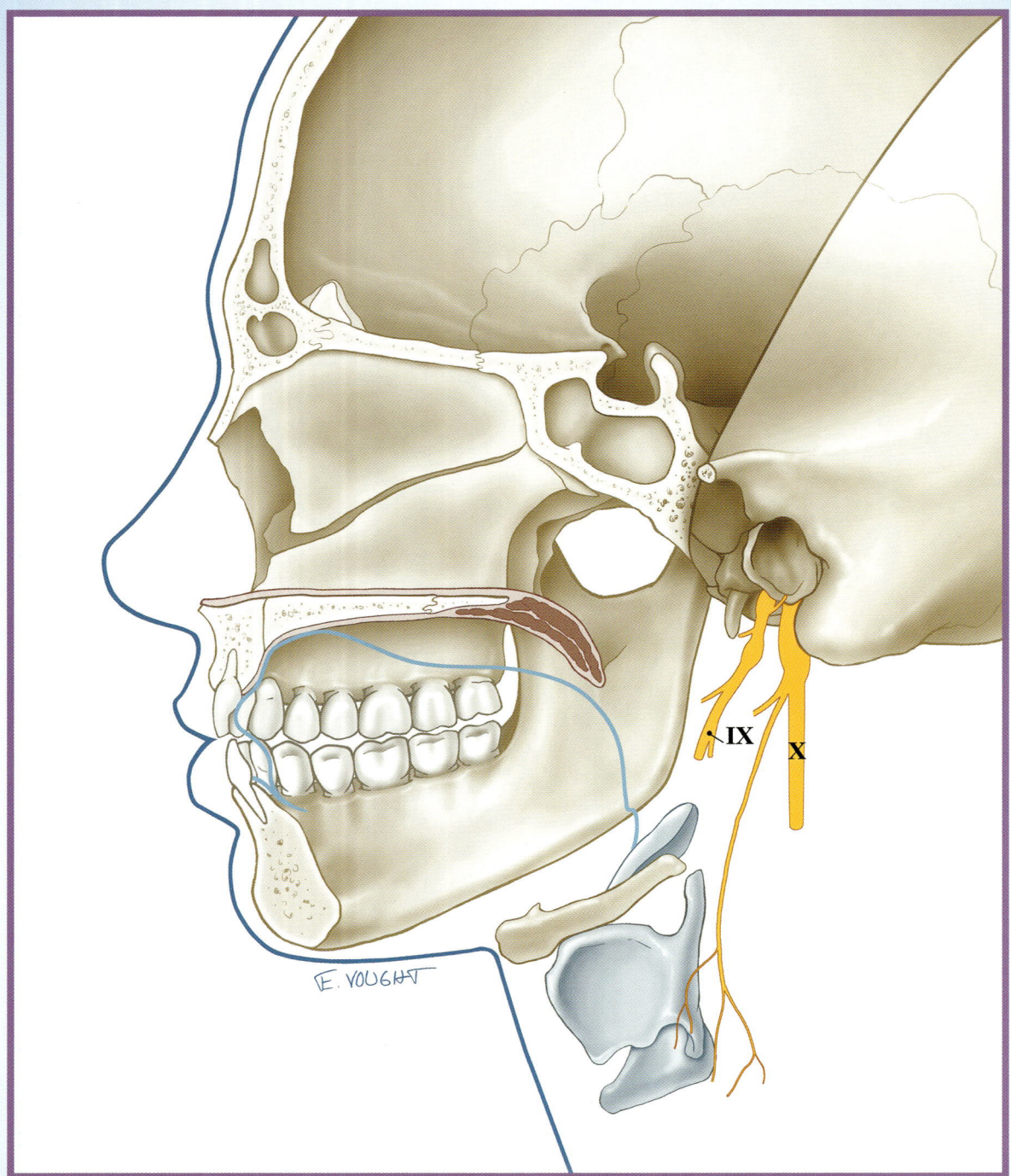

Figure 12 Cranial nerves associated with Component 6 – Initiation of Pharyngeal Swallow.
IX and X refer to glossopharyngeal and vagus nerves, respectively.

Pharyngeal Domain
Component 7 – Soft Palate Elevation (and Retraction)

In a lateral 2-D videofluorographic image as observed on a MBSS, the soft palate engages in a progressive elevation and retraction movement to contact the posterior pharyngeal wall (i.e., the anteriorly displaced superior pharyngeal constrictor). The complete contact of the soft palate to the posterior (and lateral) pharyngeal wall prevents retrograde flow of the bolus into the nasopharynx. A strong composite pressure is developed via contact of the soft palate, pharyngeal walls, and base of tongue that drives the bolus through the pharyngeal cavity facilitating complete clearance of the bolus through the pharynx.

Table 7 Muscles associated with MBSImP Component 7 – Soft Palate Elevation			
Functional Group	**Name**	**Innervation**	**Action**
Muscles of the soft palate	**Levator veli palatini**	CN X	Elevates, tenses, and retracts the soft palate against the posterior pharyngeal wall
	Tensor veli palatini	CN V	
	Musculus uvulae	CN X	

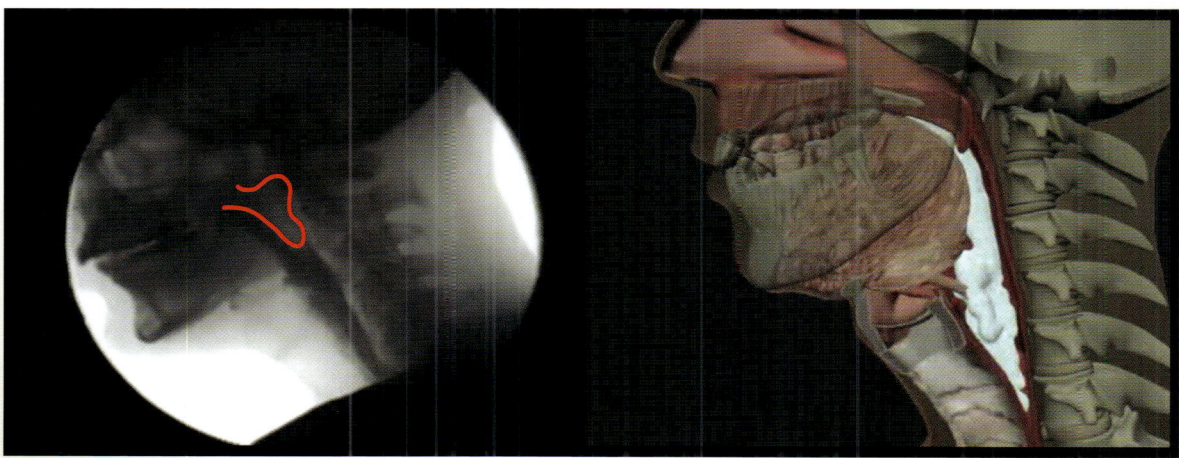

Figure 13 Videofluoroscopic and 3-D animated images demonstrating Component 7 – Soft Palate Elevation.

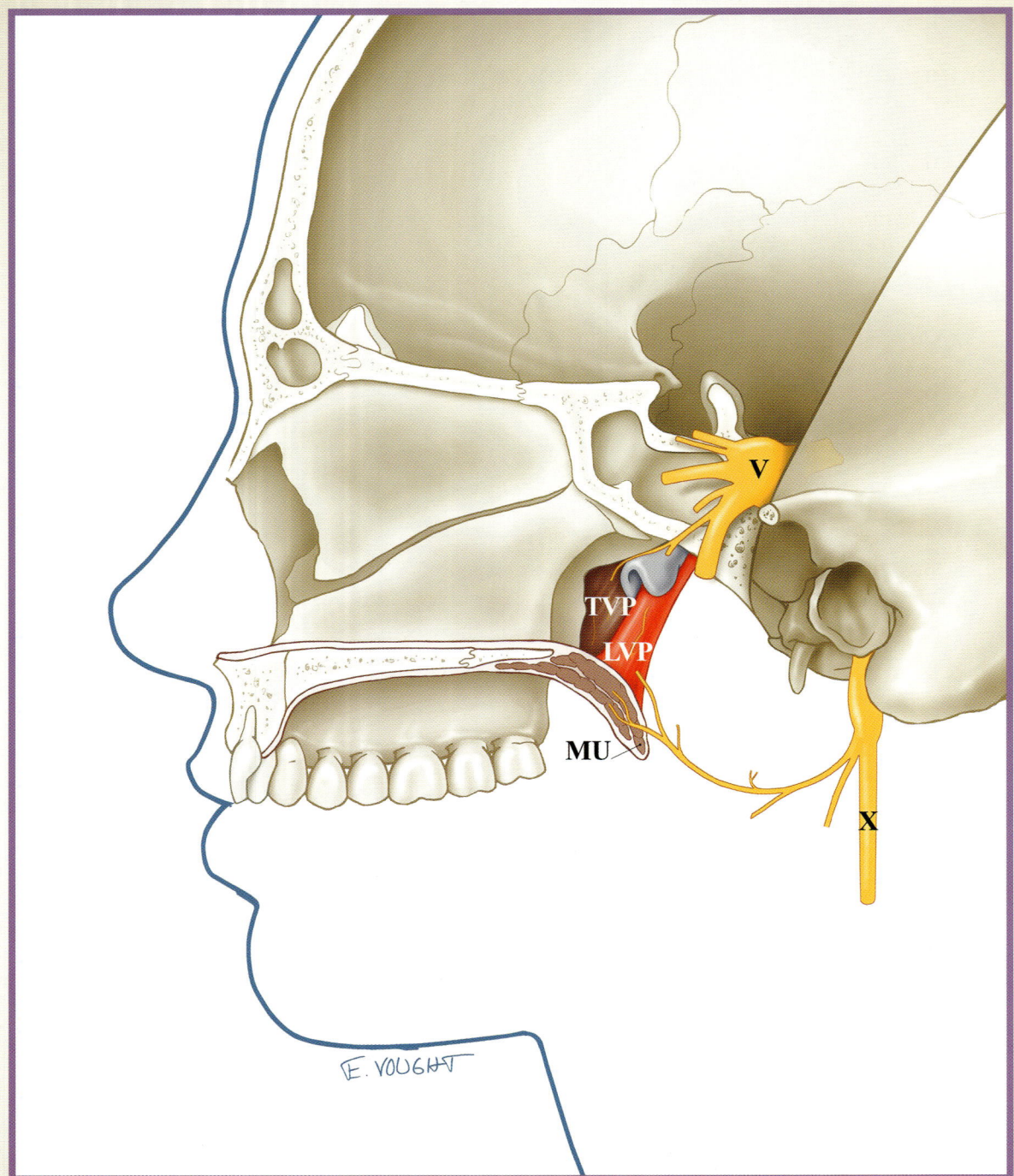

Figure 14 Muscles and innervation of Component 7 – Soft Palate Elevation. LVP-Levator veli palatini; MU-Musculus uvulae; TVP-Tensor veli palatini. V and X refer to trigeminal and vagus nerves, respectively.

Pharyngeal Domain
Component 8 – Laryngeal Elevation

Elevation of the larynx is accomplished by contraction (shortening) of the thyrohyoid muscle. Past and recent works also lend support to the influence of pharyngeal muscle contraction (shortening) on elevation of the larynx because of the nature and location of the insertion of the pharyngeal muscles onto the laryngeal cartilage. Clinical evidence provided from known pharyngeal muscle injury induced by radiation or surgery and the respective negative influence on laryngeal elevation also supports this anatomic and physiologic theory. Therefore, observations of laryngeal elevation viewed on the lateral videofluoroscopic image provide indirect information regarding the ability of the pharynx to shorten.

Years of clinical and research experience demonstrate that it is not possible to formulate reliable or meaningful visual judgments of the degree of laryngeal elevation from videofluoroscopic images between patients or groups of dysphagic patients. The functional result of laryngeal elevation is displacement of the epiglottis to a horizontal position (the first step toward full inversion) that shields the laryngeal inlet and accentuates the epiglottic petiole (base). Laryngeal elevation also facilitates a downward, inward, and forward displacement of the arytenoid cartilages that contact the epiglottic petiole. Together these mechanisms serve to shield the laryngeal inlet from ingested material passing through the pharynx. Therefore, the functional result of laryngeal elevation (i.e., the degree of contact between the arytenoid cartilage(s) and the epiglottic petiole at the time of horizontal displacement of the body of the epiglottis) is used as a surrogate indicator for judging the integrity of laryngeal elevation. In summary, the first line of airway protection, arytenoid-to-epiglottic base contact that occurs during normal laryngeal elevation, is the determinant used for judging adequate laryngeal elevation rather than attempting time intensive, discrete distance measurements that have not been rigorously tested for their clinical validity.

Table 8 Muscles associated with MBSImP Component 8 – Laryngeal Elevation

Functional Group	Name	Innervation	Action
Long pharyngeal muscles	**Stylopharyngeus**	CN IX	Shortens and widens the pharynx
	Salpingopharyngeus	CN X	
	Palatopharyngeus		Elevates the larynx*
Infrahyoid muscle	**Thyrohyoid**	C1	Elevates the thyroid cartilage to the hyoid
Intrinsic muscles of the larynx	Thyroarytenoid	CN X	Downward, inward, and forward rotation and approximation of the arytenoid cartilages to meet bulging epiglottic petiole
	Lateral cricoarytenoid		
	Interarytenoid		Adducts (closes) the true vocal folds and approximation of the ventricular folds

*Elevation of larynx displaces epiglottis to horizontal position.

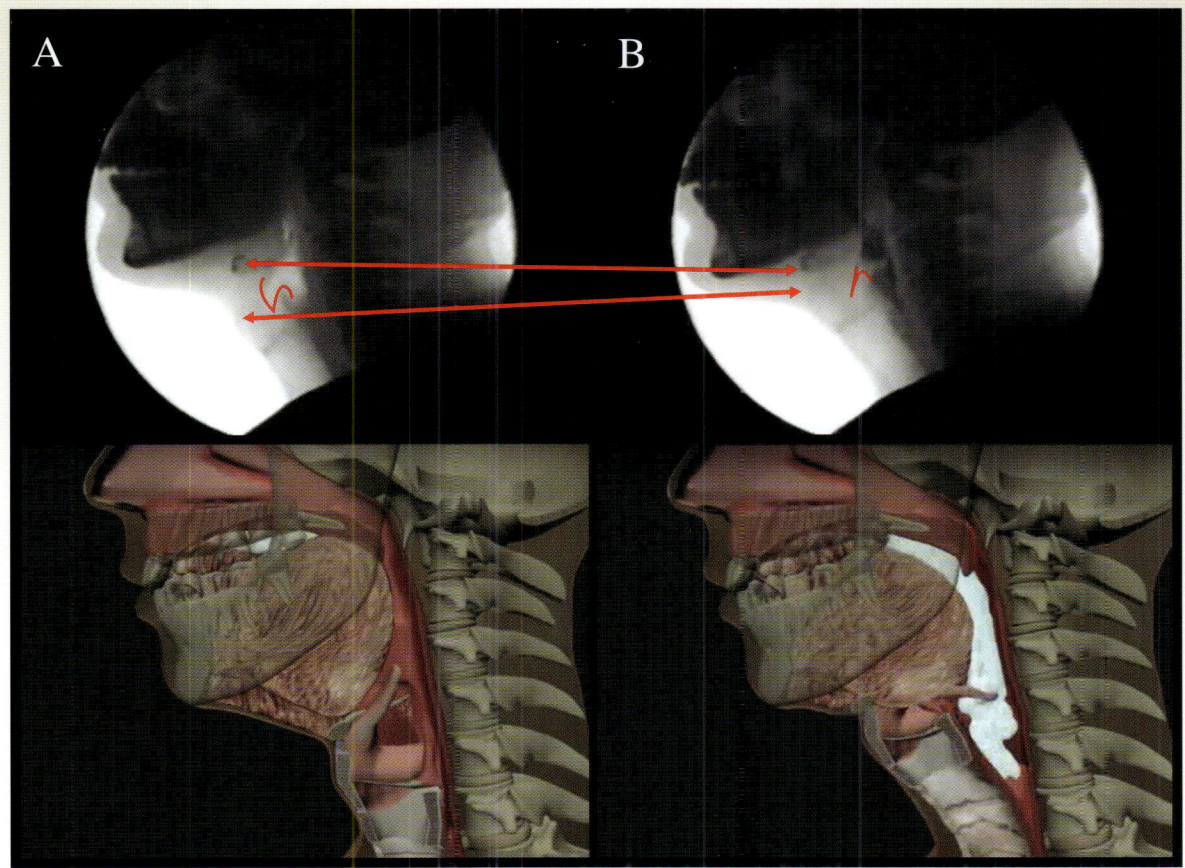

Figure 15 Videofluoroscopic and 3-D animated images demonstrating Component 8 – Laryngeal Elevation. (A) Hyoid and larynx at rest. (B) Maximal displacement of hyoid and larynx.

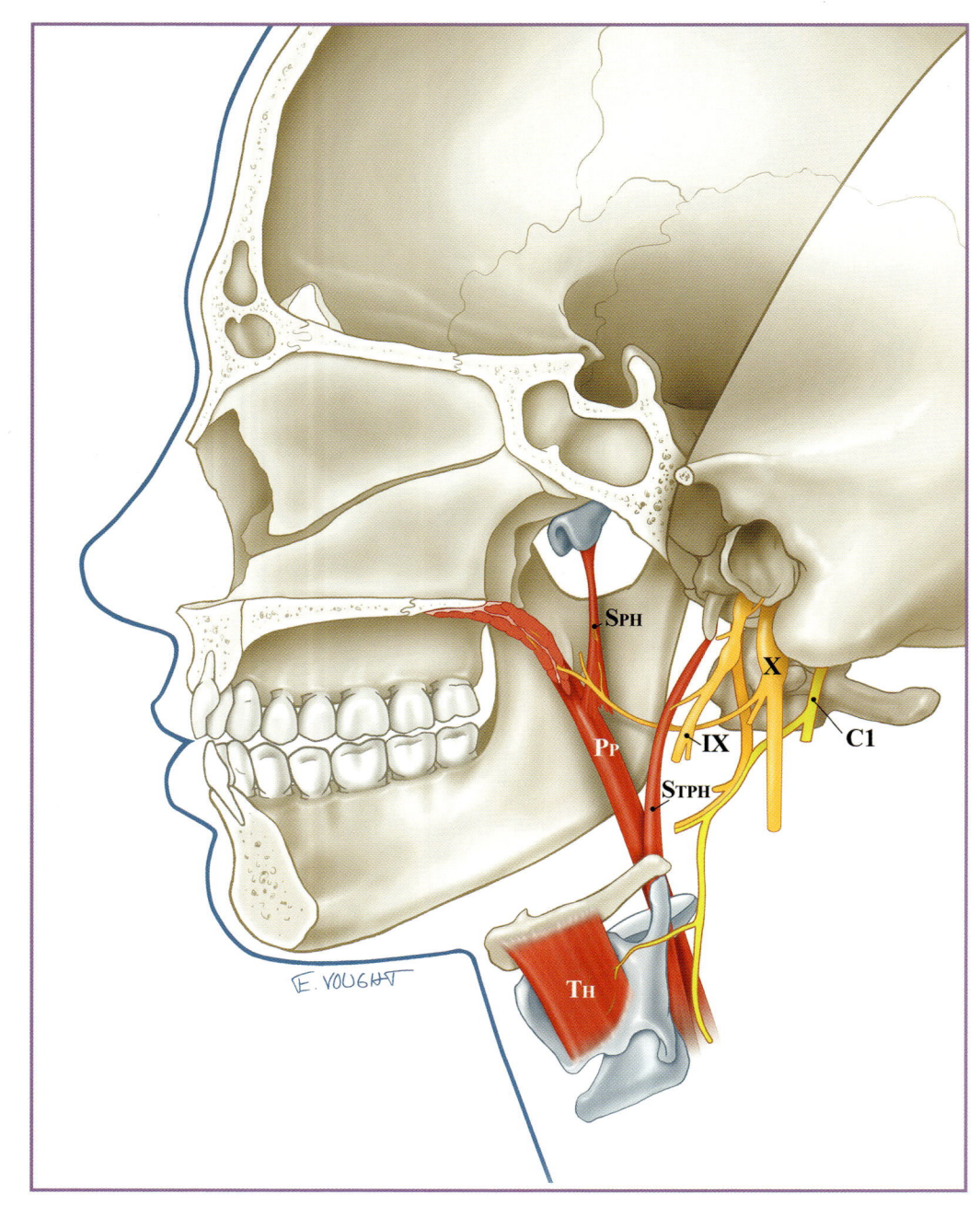

Figure 16 Muscles and innervation of Component 8 – Laryngeal Elevation. I-Interarytenoid; LC-Lateral cricoarytenoid; Pp-Palatopharyngeus; Sph-Salpingopharyngeus; Stph-Stylopharyngeus;

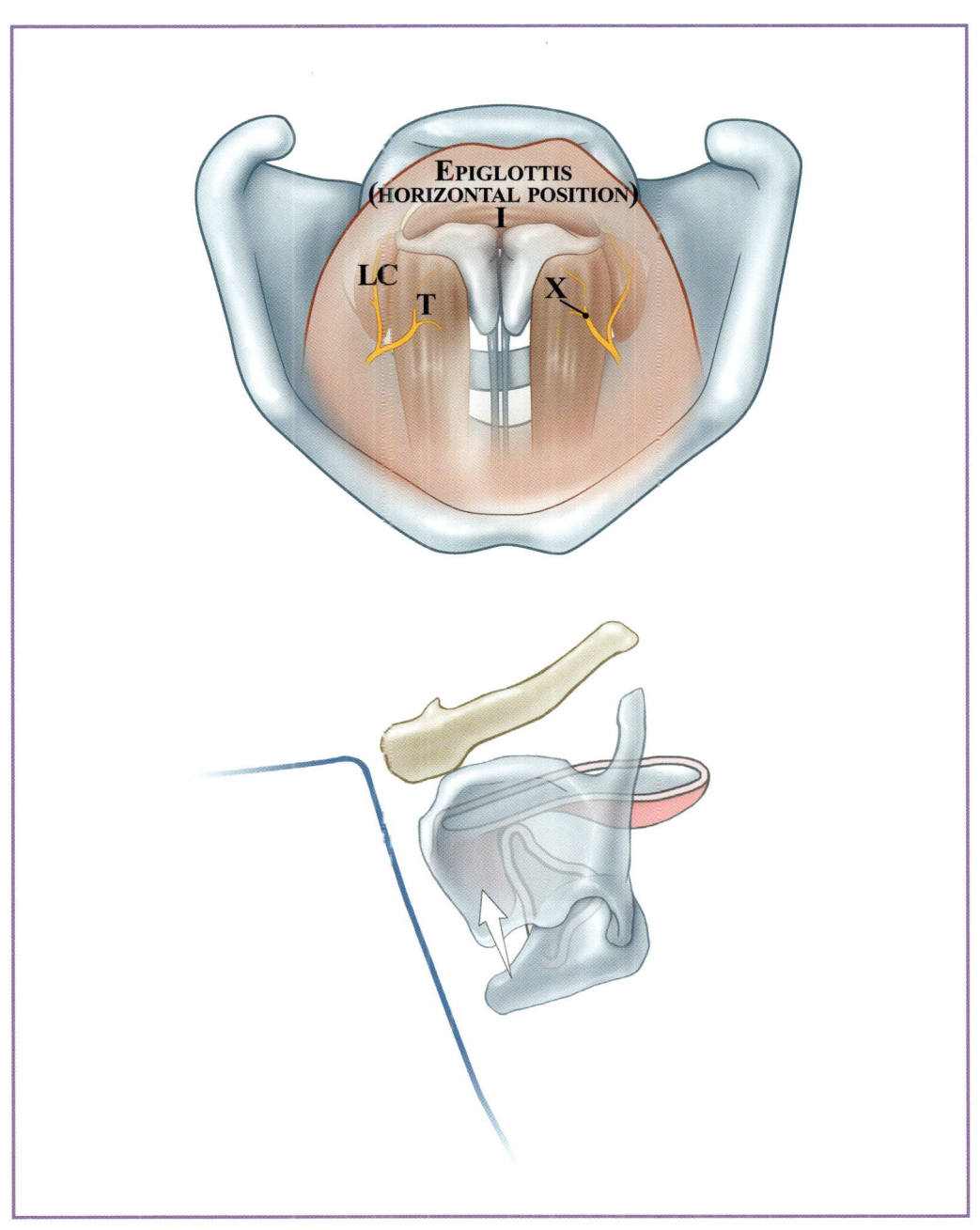

T-Thyroarytenoid; TH-Thyrohyoid. X and X refer to glossopharyngeal and vagus nerves, respectively. C1 refers to cervical spinal nerve 1.

Pharyngeal Domain
Component 9 – Anterior Hyoid Excursion

The association between the most extreme anterior hyoid movement (signaling the height of the pharyngeal swallow) and opening of the PES is well established. Further, complete (inferior) inversion of the epiglottis (Component 10) has been attributed to traction placed by anterior hyoid displacement during swallowing. The hyoid is intimately (anatomically) connected to the thyroid cartilage and thus, they are often referred to as a functional unit; i.e., the hyolaryngeal complex.

Similar to visual perceptual judgments of laryngeal elevation, reliable and valid measures of hyoid displacement during a MBSS are time intensive, subject to poor reliability, and have not been tested for their clinical validity. The MBSImP approach has informed us that visual perceptual judgment of the angle of the thyroid cartilage relative to the position of the hyoid bone represents a reliable indicator of the integrity of anterior hyoid motion. In cases of complete anterior hyoid motion, the angle of trajectory is more acute (visually 45° or less). When the anterior movement of the hyoid is incomplete, the laryngeal cartilage is in more of a direct line with the hyoid bone (greater than 45° but less than 90°). Although anterior hyoid movement has been implicated as the primary player in PESO, we and others using the MBSImP metrics have observed dysphagic patients to open the PES (at least to functional levels for passage of liquids and semisolids) with no evidence of anterior hyoid movement. These dysphagic patients demonstrate the capability to generate compensatory or adaptive contractions of the pharynx that may play a role in PESO in patients with impaired anterior hyoid movement, although the mechanisms are not understood.

Table 9 Muscles associated with MBSImP Component 9 – Anterior Hyoid Excursion

Functional Group	Name	Innervation	Action
Suprahyoid muscles	**Geniohyoid**	CN 1	Anterior movement of the hyoid
	Mylohyoid	CN V	
	Digastricus	Anterior belly: CN V	

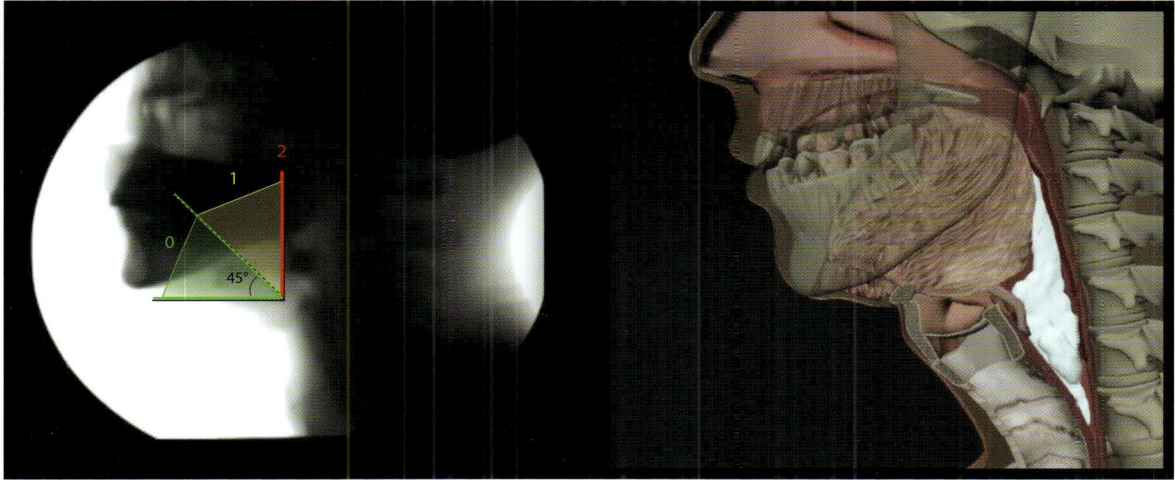

Figure 17 Videofluoroscopic and 3-D animated images demonstrating Component 9 – Anterior Hyoid Excursion.

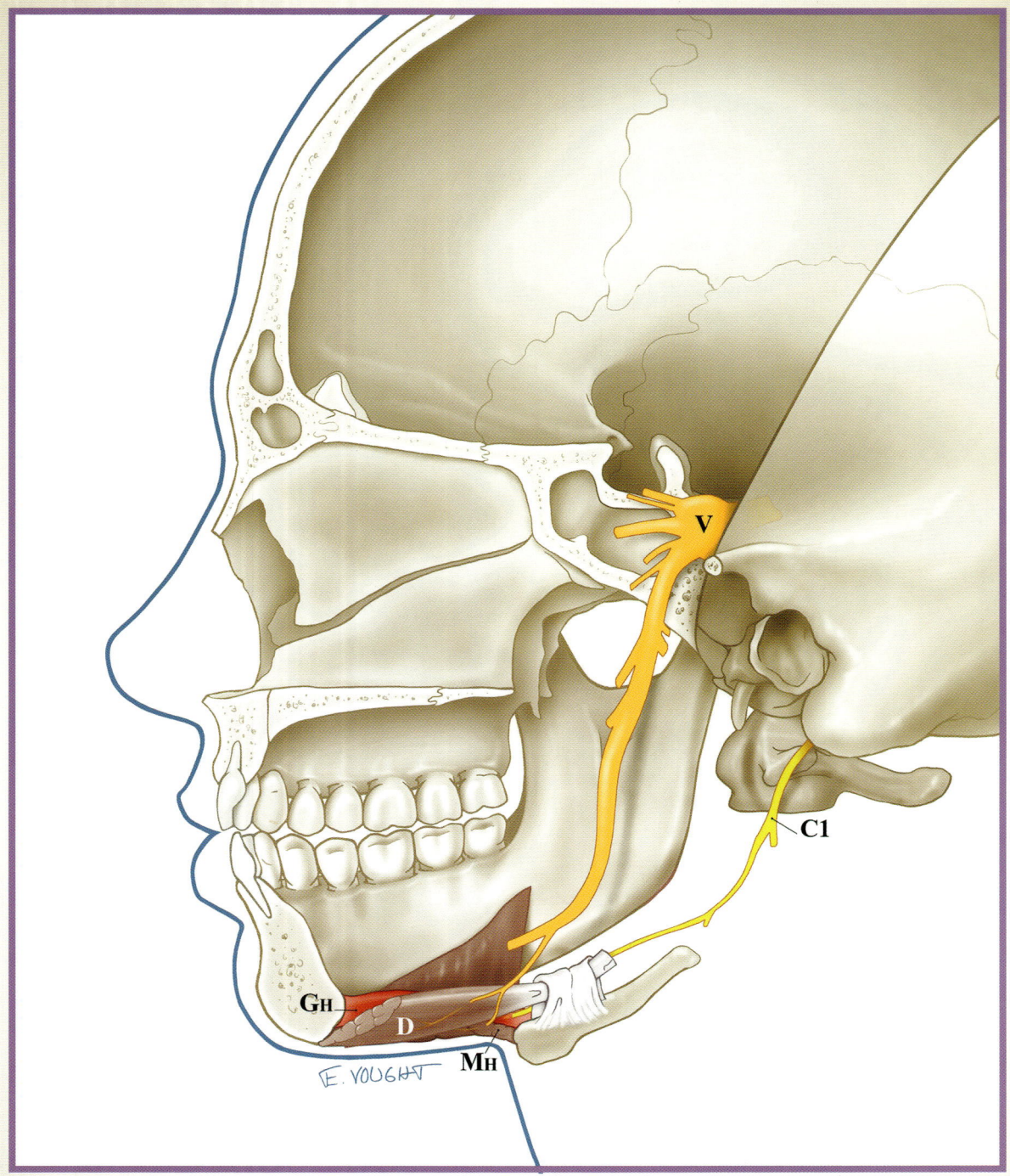

Figure 18 Muscles and innervation of Component 9 – Anterior Hyoid Excursion. D-Digastricus; GH-Geniohyoid; MH-Mylohyoid. V refers to trigeminal nerve. C1 refers to cervical spinal nerve 1.

Pharyngeal Domain
Component 10 – Epiglottic Movement (Inversion)

The epiglottis is a rigid cartilage and represents the uppermost structure of the larynx. At rest, the epiglottis has no known functional relevance. During the act of swallowing, the epiglottis engages in a two-stage process of inversion to assist in timing bolus flow and protecting the laryngeal inlet as the bolus passes through the pharynx. The first stage of epiglottic inversion is achieved by laryngeal elevation (Component 8). (There is some mention of contribution by a thyroepiglottic muscle, but the presence and function of this structure remains unclear.) Elevation of the larynx displaces the epiglottis to a horizontal position in healthy, non-dysphagic adults. The second stage of inversion, complete inferior displacement, is achieved primarily by anterior traction of the hyolaryngeal complex. The literature and clinical observations also implicate the retraction of the tongue base and its contact to the anteriorly displaced (middle) pharyngeal wall. These latter mechanisms appear to be most functionally relevant in dysphagic patients who have impaired anterior hyoid (hyolaryngeal) movement (Component 9). Patients can be trained (by self or in treatment) to exaggerate the contraction of the tongue base and posterior pharyngeal wall, presumably leading to increased pressure that assists in epiglottic inversion when hyoid movement is reduced or absent.

Table 10 Muscles associated with MBSImP Component 10 – Epiglottic Movement

Functional Group	Name	Innervation	Action
Suprahyoid muscles	**Geniohyoid**	C 1	Elevates and moves the hyoid anteriorly contributing to superior-anterior movement trajectory
	Mylohyoid	CN V	
	Digastricus	Anterior belly: CN V	
Muscles of the base of tongue	Hyoglossus	CN XII	Retracts the base of tongue
	Styloglossus		
	Palatoglossus	CN X	
	Middle pharyngeal constrictor		Supports other action of muscles listed here, including laryngeal elevation and tongue base to posterior pharyngeal wall contact
Long pharyngeal muscles	Palatopharyngeus	CN X	Shortens and widens the pharynx
	Salpingopharyngeus		
	Stylopharyngeus	CN IX	Elevates the larynx*
Infrahyoid muscle	Thyrohyoid	C1	Elevates the thyroid cartilage to the hyoid

*Elevation of larynx displaces epiglottis to horizontal position.

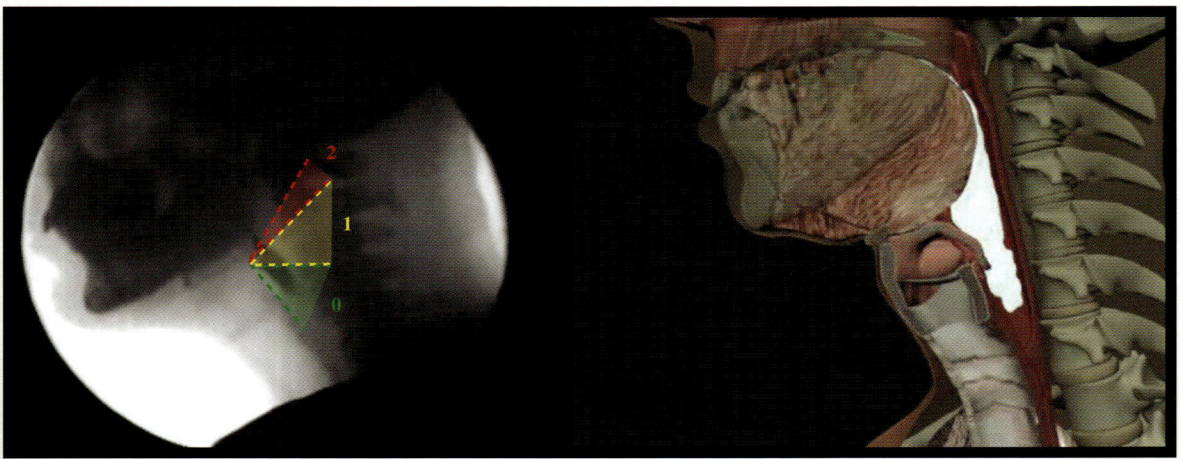

Figure 19 Videofluoroscopic and 3-D animated images demonstrating Component 10 – Epiglottic Movement.

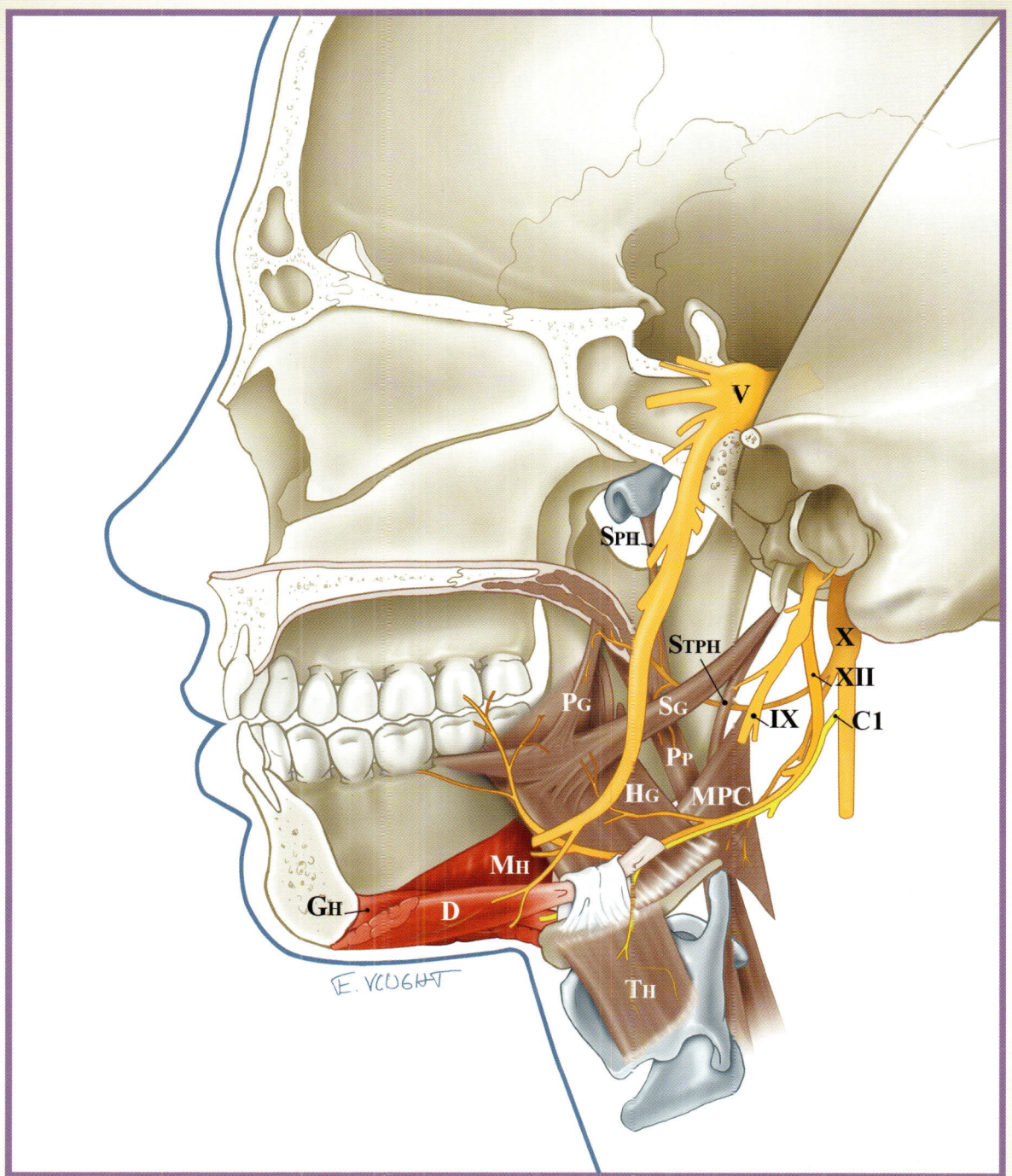

Figure 20 Muscles and innervation of Component 10 – Epiglottic Movement. D-Digastricus (anterior belly); GH-Geniohyoid; HG-Hyoglossus; MH-Mylohyoid; MPC-Middle pharyngeal constrictor; PG-Palatoglossus; PP-Palatopharyngeus; SG-Styloglossus; SPH-Salpingopharyngeus; STPH-Stylopharyngeus; TH-Thyrohyoid. V, IX, X, and XII refer to trigeminal, glossopharyngeal, vagus, and hypoglossal nerves, respectively. C1 refers to the cervical spinal nerve 1.

Pharyngeal Domain
Component 11 – Laryngeal Vestibular Closure (Height of Swallow)

Whereas early closure of the laryngeal inlet occurs during laryngeal elevation (Component 8), late laryngeal vestibular closure occurs at the height of anterior hyoid (hyolaryngeal) displacement (Component 9). The laryngeal vestibule is tightly sealed at this time via intrinsic laryngeal structures, including true vocal folds and ventricular folds (not directly observed in the lateral fluoroscopic plane), and extrinsic mechanisms, such as full inversion of the epiglottis (Component 10) and retraction of the tongue base (Component 15) with contact to the anteriorly displaced posterior pharyngeal wall (Component 12). Clinical evidence supports patients may have intact early laryngeal vestibular closure because of adequate laryngeal elevation (Score of (0) on Component 8 – complete approximation of the arytenoid cartilages to the epiglottic petiole) as the epiglottis inverts to a horizontal position; however, lack of complete anterior hyolaryngeal motion will result in various degrees of impairment in late laryngeal vestibular closure, including incomplete inversion of the epiglottis.

Table 11 Muscles associated with MBSImP Component 11 – Laryngeal Vestibular Closure

Functional Group	Name	Innervation	Action
Intrinsic muscles of the larynx	Thyroarytenoid	CN X	Downward, inward, and forward rotation and approximation of the arytenoid cartilages to meet bulging epiglottic petiole associated with laryngeal elevation (Component 8-Laryngeal Elevation)
	Lateral cricoarytenoid		
	Interarytenoid		Adducts (closes) the true vocal folds and approximation of ventricular folds
Muscles of the base of tongue	Styloglossus	CN XII	Retracts the base of tongue and assists in shielding laryngeal inlet
	Palatoglossus	CN X	

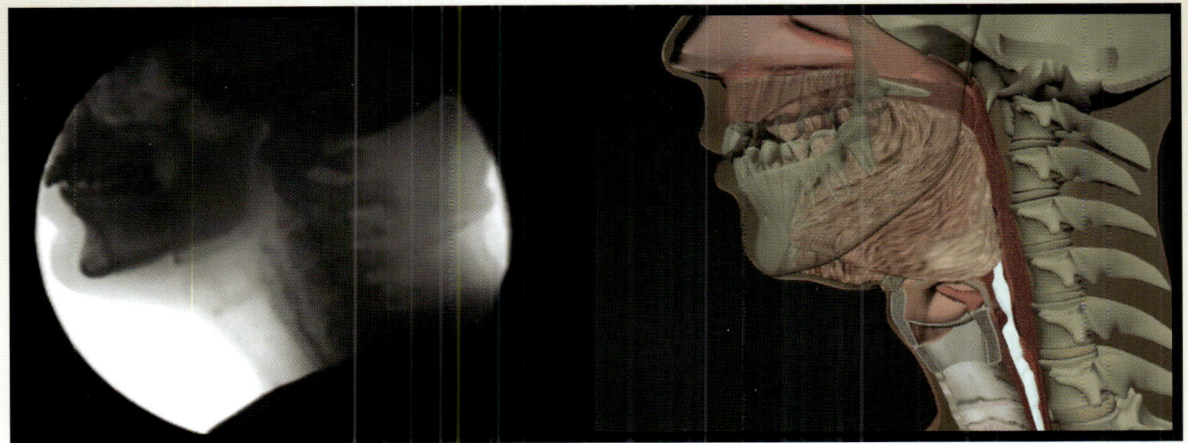

Figure 21 Videofluoroscopic and 3-D animated images demonstrating Component 11 – Laryngeal Vestibular Closure-Height of Swallow.

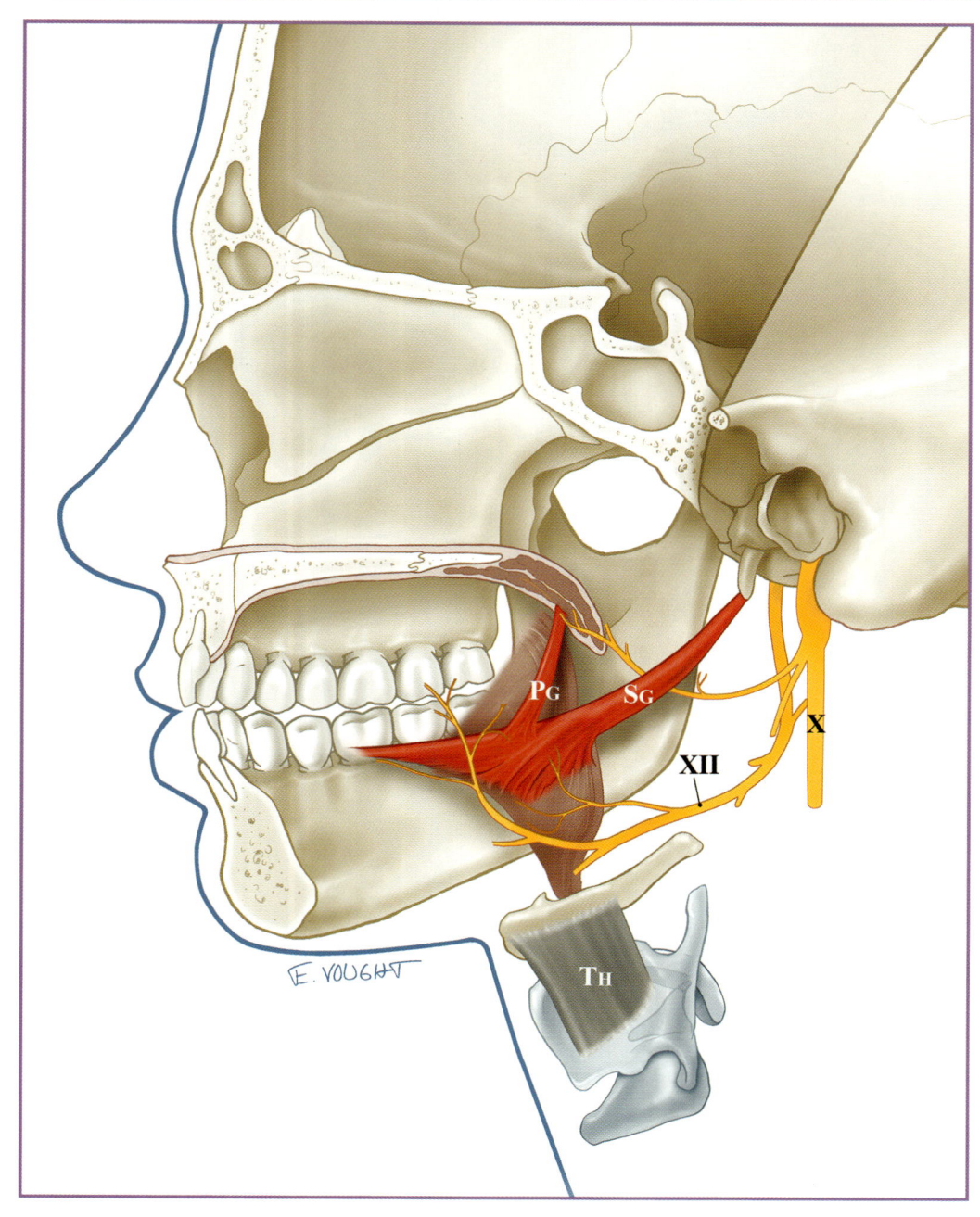

Figure 22 Muscles and innervation of Component 11 – Laryngeal Vestibular Closure-Height of Swallow. I-Interarytenoid; LC-Lateral cricoarytenoid; PG-Palatoglossus; SG-Styloglossus;

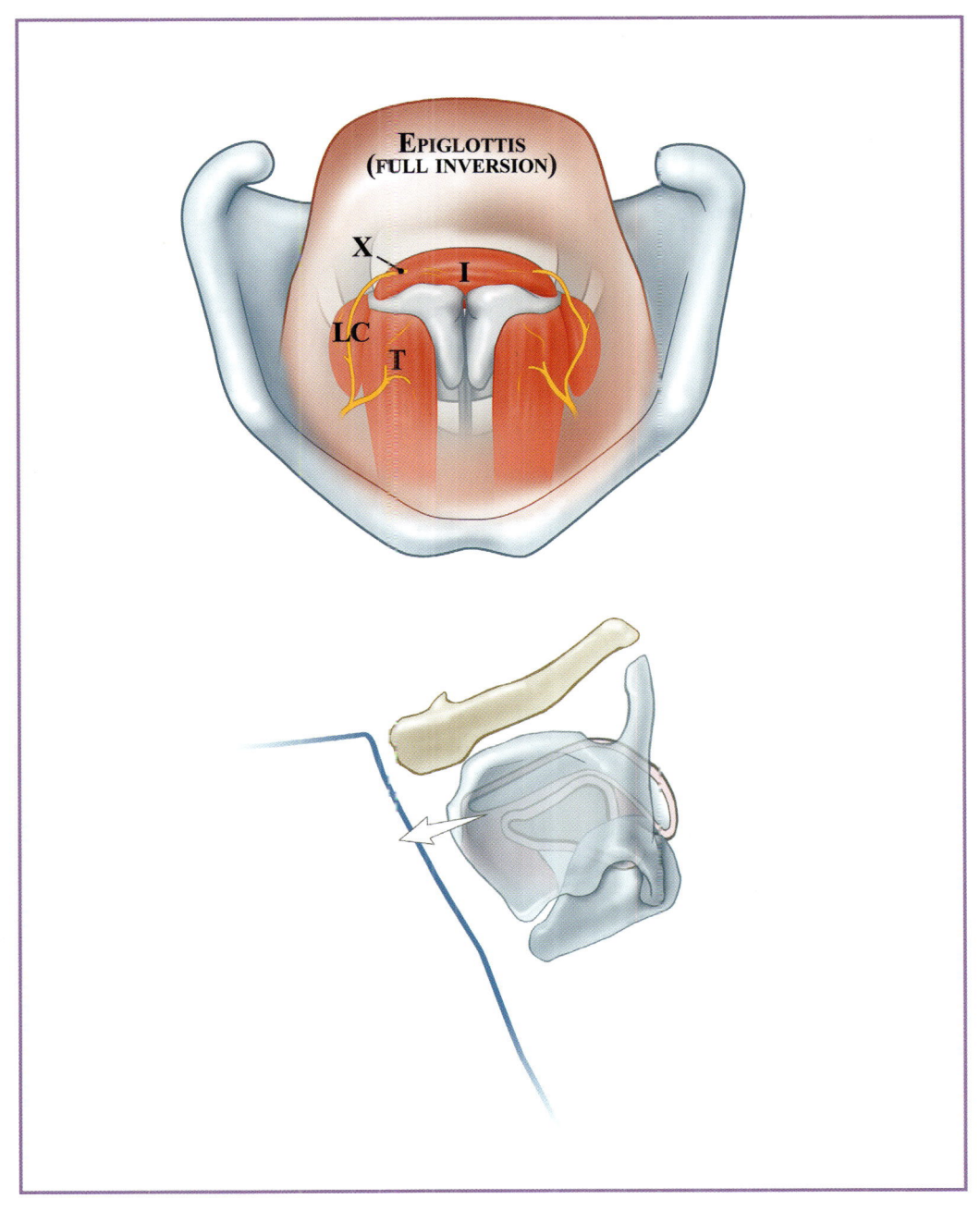

T-Thyroarytenoid; TH-Thyrohyoid (illustrated for role in early laryngeal vestibular closure - Component 8, Laryngeal Elevation). X and XII refer to vagus and hypoglossal nerves, respectively.

Pharyngeal Domain
Component 12 – Pharyngeal Stripping Wave

The stripping action of the pharynx is achieved by sequential, progressive contraction of the superior, middle, and inferior pharyngeal constrictor muscles. The stripping wave is represented by anterior bulging of the posterior pharyngeal wall superiorly to inferiorly and ends with closure of the PES as the pharynx and larynx return to rest. Once thought insignificant as a propulsive force against the bolus tail, new evidence points to its potentially critical role in assisting pharyngeal clearance through its composite pressure generation with the tongue base and potentially soft palate. Dysphagic patients have been shown to develop large, exaggerated stripping wave motions to accommodate reductions in tongue base retraction. It may be the case that pharyngeal stripping is far more significant to efficient bolus passage in dysphagic patients who have compromised tongue base motion. If the stripping wave is diminished or absent, but without any other oropharyngeal impairments, the functional result will be only a lining of contrast material on the posterior pharyngeal wall after initial swallow completion. Pharyngeal residue (Component 16) may be present when decreased or absent pharyngeal stripping is accompanied by a reduction in tongue base retraction resulting in a collection or majority of contrast remaining in the pharyngeal recesses.

Table 12 Muscles associated with MBSImP Component 12 – Pharyngeal Stripping Wave

Functional Group	Name	Innervation	Action
Pharyngeal constrictor muscles	Superior constrictor	CN X	Applies positive pressure generation to the bolus tail through sequential contractions superiorly to inferiorly
	Middle constrictor		
	Inferior constrictor		

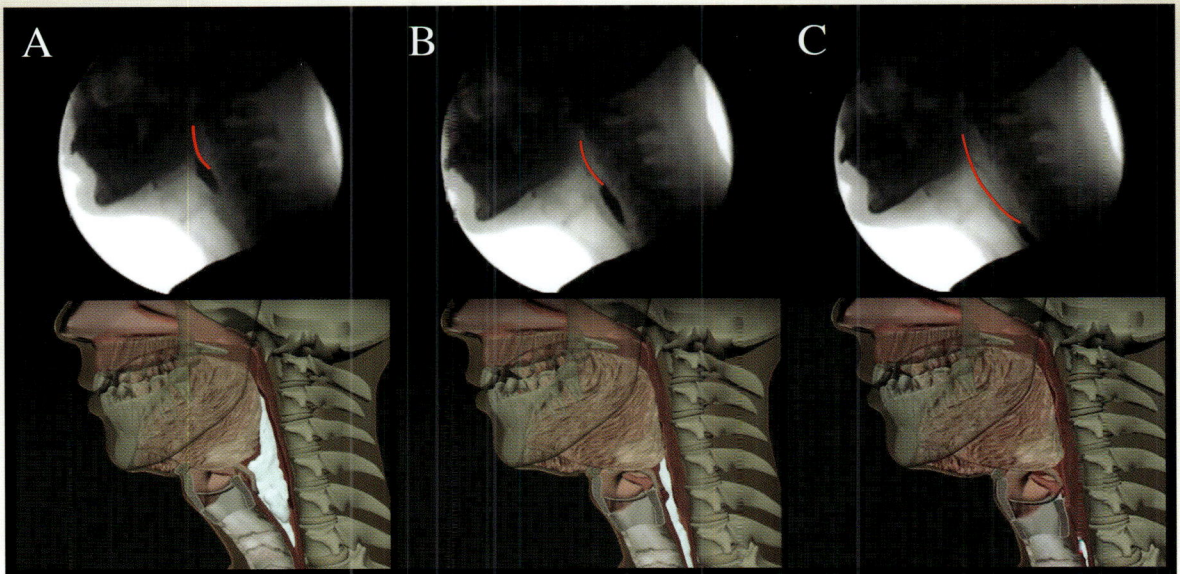

Figure 23 Videofluoroscopic and 3-D animated images demonstrating Component 12 – Pharyngeal Stripping Wave. (A) Initiation of pharyngeal stripping wave as bolus is pushed through pharynx. (B) Continuation of pharyngeal stripping wave as bolus head enters cervical esophagus. (C) Completion of pharyngeal stripping wave as bolus tail enters cervical esophagus.

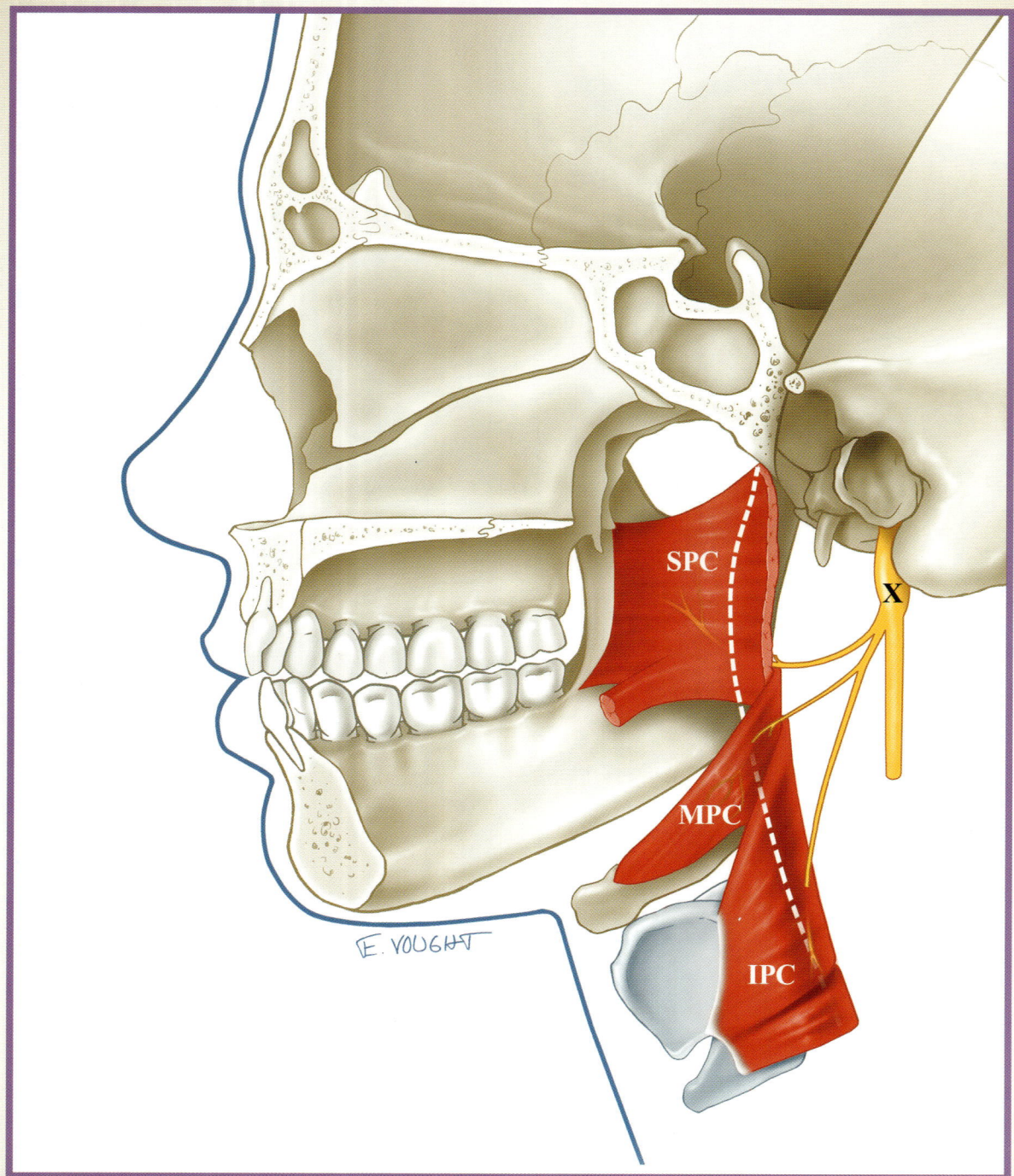

Figure 24 Muscles and innervation of Component 12 – Pharyngeal Stripping Wave. IPC-Inferior pharyngeal constrictor; MPC-Middle pharyngeal constrictor; SPC-Superior pharyngeal constrictor. X refers to vagus nerve.

Pharyngeal Domain
Component 13 – Pharyngeal Contraction (A/P View)

Pharyngeal contraction is the combined action of pharyngeal shortening (indirectly observed during laryngeal elevation, Component 8) and pharyngeal stripping (Component 12), and it is observed in A/P fluoroscopic viewing plane. The patient should be positioned with the head in the upright, neutral position whenever possible to achieve full viewing of the pharynx, larynx, and cervical esophagus (PES region). Careful viewing of the swallow will reveal shortening (lifting) of the pharynx as the head of the bolus enters the pharynx after the onset of the pharyngeal swallow (Component 6). During this time, the larynx is elevating (Component 8), and the examiner can occasionally view the epiglottis in a horizontal position in A/P viewing plane. Attention should focus on the superior to inferior compression of the pharyngeal walls (pharyngeal stripping in the lateral view, Component 12) on the bolus tail as the bolus clears the pharynx, and enters and passes through the PES.

Table 13 Muscles associated with MBSImP Component 13 – Pharyngeal Contraction
(combination of shortening and stripping viewed in the A/P viewing plane)

Functional Group	Name	Innervation	Action
Pharyngeal constrictor muscles	Superior constrictor	CN X	Applies positive pressure generation to the bolus tail through sequential contractions superiorly to inferiorly
	Middle constrictor		
	Inferior constrictor		
Long pharyngeal muscles	Stylopharyngeus	CN IX	Shortens and widens the pharynx
	Salpingopharyngeus	CN X	Elevates the larynx*
	Palatopharyngeus		

*Elevation of larynx displaces epiglottis to horizontal position.

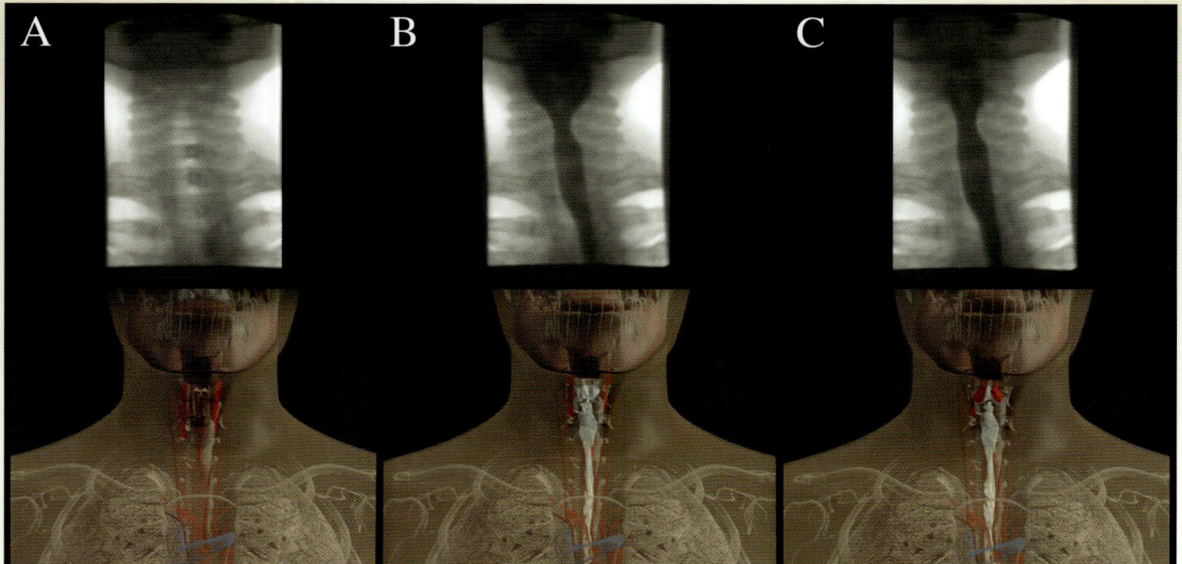

Figure 25 Videofluoroscopic and 3-D animated images demonstrating Component 13 – Pharyngeal Contraction-A/P View. (A) Pharynx at rest prior to initiation of the swallow. **(B)** Bolus passes through the PES and into the esophagus as the larynx elevates and the pharynx shortens. **(C)** Complete pharyngeal contraction.as indicated by symmetrical lateral compression of pharyngeal walls against the bolus tail.

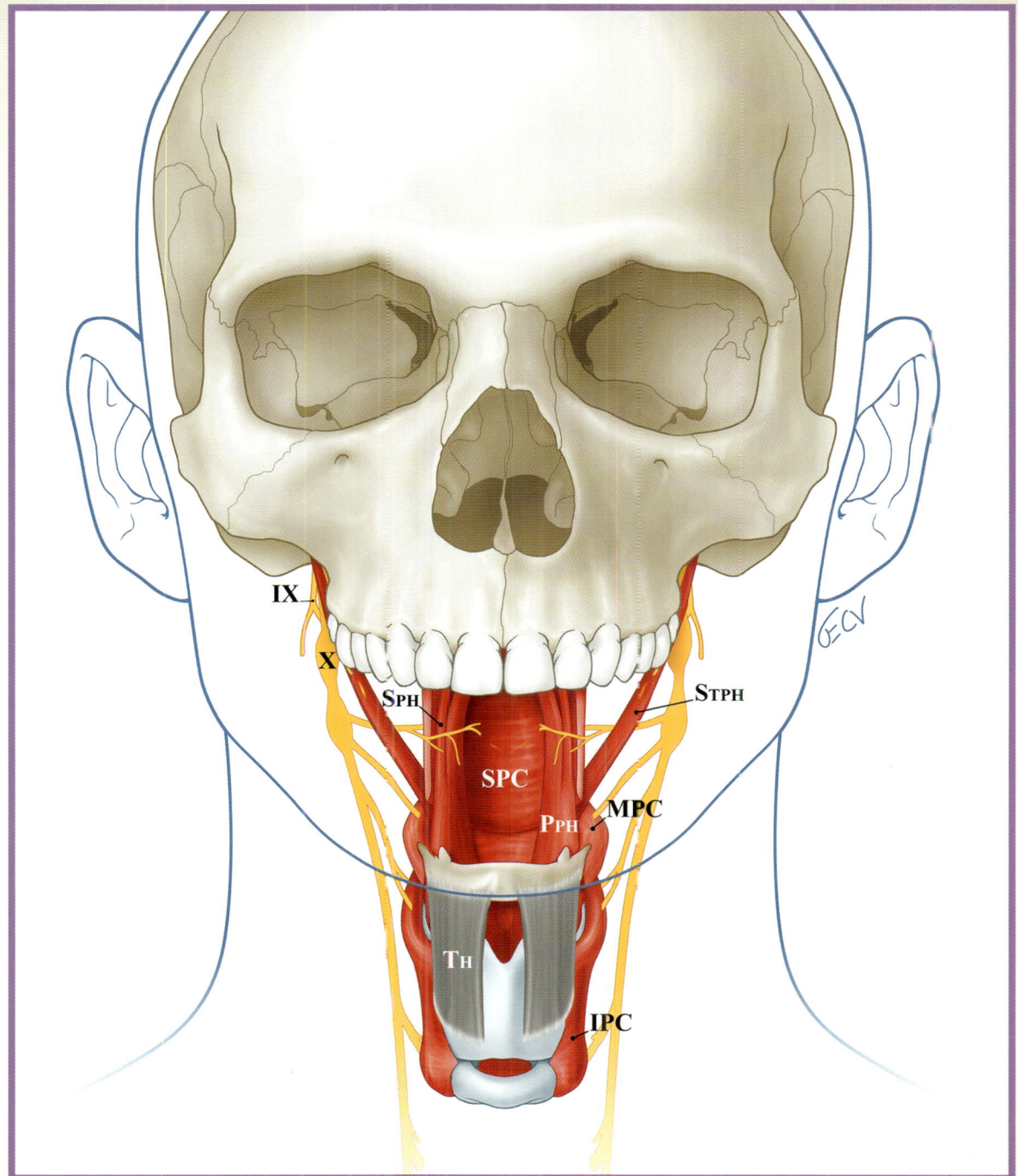

Figure 26 Muscles and innervation of Component 13 – Pharyngeal Contraction.
IPC-Inferior pharyngeal constrictor; MPC-Middle pharyngeal constrictor; PPH-Palatopharyngeus; SPH-Salpingopharyngeus; STPH-Stylopharyngeus; SPC-Superior pharyngeal constrictor; TH-Thyrohyoid (illustrated for role in laryngeal elevation (Component 8) that occurs simultaneously with pharyngeal shortening). IX and X refer to glossopharyngeal and vagus nerves, respectively.

Pharyngeal Domain
Component 14 – Pharyngoesophageal Segment Opening

The PES is comprised of the cricopharyngeus muscle (CPM), fibers of the inferior constrictor muscle, and tight approximation of the cricoid cartilage against the posterior pharyngeal wall. The CPM is tonically contracted at rest to prevent ingestion of air during respiration and regurgitation of material from the stomach and esophagus. It relaxes at the onset of the pharyngeal swallow via motor command from the vagus nerve. This relaxation does not open the PES, but rather results in a compliant muscle that facilitates opening through biomechanical forces applied by the hyolaryngeal complex and potentially the pharynx. As the hyoid and larynx proceed as a functional unit in an upward forward trajectory, the cricoid cartilage is pulled away from the posterior pharyngeal wall. This combination of traction forces and CPM relaxation leads to complete distention of the PES as observed by a fairly symmetrical tube without indentation or obstruction to bolus flow. Any disruptions in the traction forces that serve to open the PES may not only interfere with complete distension of the segment, but may also result in shortening the duration of PESO. Complete PESO with incomplete distension will result in cutting off a portion of the bolus prior to complete passage into the esophagus. The functional implication will be retention of contrast in the pyriform sinuses and higher (worse) scores for Component 16 (Pharyngeal Residue).

Table 14 Muscles associated with MBSImP Component 14 – Pharyngoesophageal Segment Opening

Functional Group	Name	Innervation	Action
Pharyngoesophageal segment (PES)	**Cricopharyngeus**	CN X	Tonically contracted at rest but relaxes during swallowing to facilitate bolus passage
	Inferior pharyngeal constrictor	CN X	Functional component of the PES region
Suprahyoid muscles	Digastricus	Anterior belly: CN V	Elevates and moves the hyoid in a superior-anterior movement trajectory pulling cricoid away from posterior pharyngeal wall
	Geniohyoid	C1	
	Mylohyoid	CN V	
	Stylohyoid*	CN VII	
Long pharyngeal muscles	Stylopharyngeus	CN IX	Shortens the pharynx and assists in elevation of the larynx
	Salpingopharyngeus	CN X	
	Palatopharyngeus		
Infrahyoid muscle	Thyrohyoid	C1	Elevates the thyroid cartilage to the hyoid

*Although the stylohyoid is not a primary contributor, it assists in hyoid elevation.

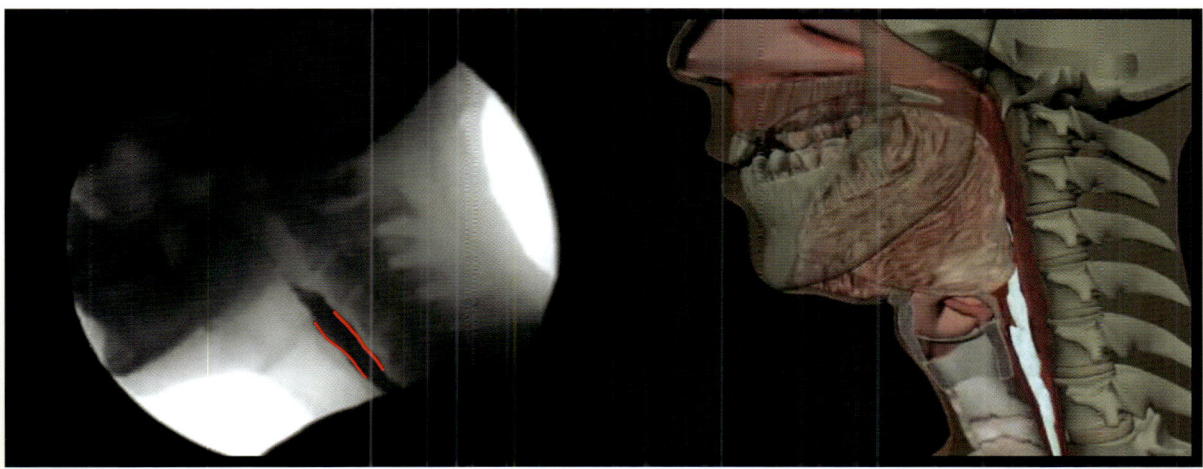

Figure 27 Videofluoroscopic and 3-D animated images demonstrating Component 14 – Pharyngoesophageal Segment Opening.

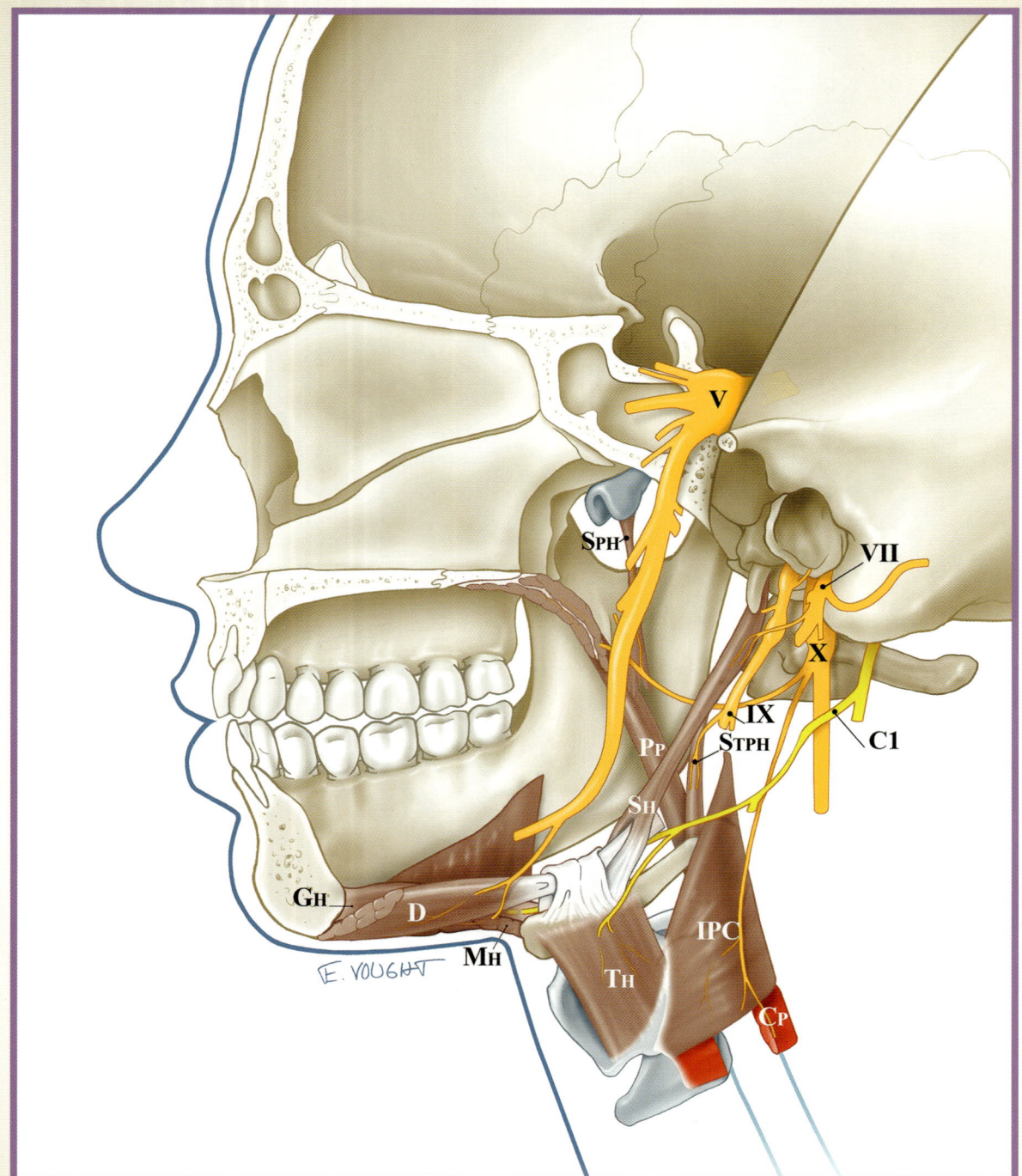

Figure 28 Muscles and innervation of Component 14 – Pharyngoesophageal Segment Opening.
Cp-Cricopharyngeus; D-Digastricus (anterior belly); Gh-Geniohyoid; IPC-Inferior pharyngeal constrictor; Mh-Mylohyoid; Pp-Palatopharyngeus; Sph-Salpingopharyngeus; Sh-Stylohyoid; Stph-Stylopharyngeus; Th-Thyrohyoid. V, VII, IX, and X refer to trigeminal, facial, glossopharyngeal, and vagus nerves, respectively. C1 refers to cervical spinal nerve 1.

Pharyngeal Domain
Component 15 – Tongue Base Retraction

Tongue base retraction has long been recognized as a primary generator of positive pressure against the bolus tail, thereby playing a critical role in pharyngeal clearance. As the tongue proceeds in a posterior direction, it assists in shielding the laryngeal inlet together with the inverting epiglottis and inward/forwardly displacing arytenoid cartilages. As a result, the tongue base is also considered a mechanism of airway protection. The base of the tongue should completely approximate the anteriorly displacing medial pharyngeal wall (Pharyngeal Stripping Wave, Component 12). If the base of tongue is the only impaired component in the dysphagic swallow, the functional results will be pharyngeal residue (Component 16) in the valleculae and on the base of tongue.

Table 15 Muscles associated with MBSImP Component 15 – Tongue Base Retraction

Functional Group	Name	Innervation	Action
Extrinsic muscles of the tongue	Styloglossus	CN XII	Retracts the base of tongue*
	Palatoglossus	CN X	
Pharyngeal constrictor	Middle pharyngeal constrictor	CN X	Constricts the middle pharynx apposing the base of tongue*

*Apposition of the base of tongue and posterior pharyngeal wall (with likely contribution of soft palate) places high composite pressure on bolus tail.

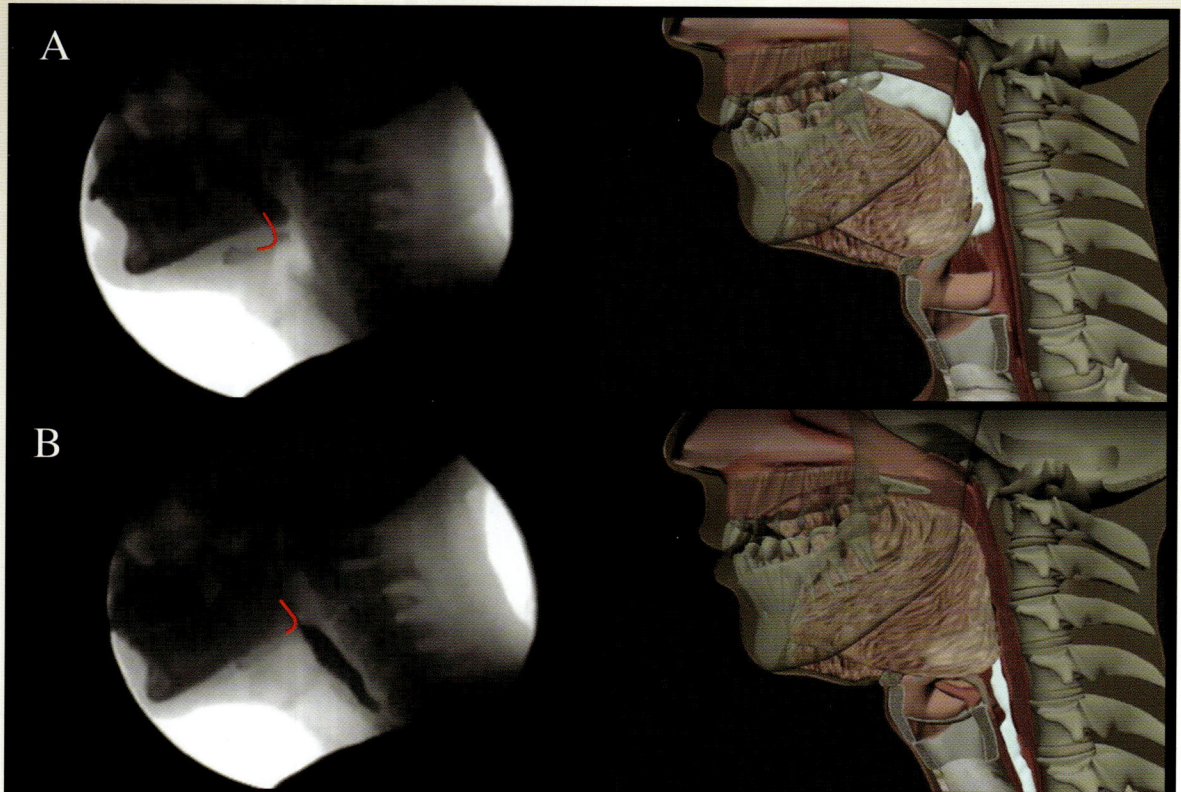

Figure 29 Videofluoroscopic and 3-D animated images demonstrating Component 15 – Tongue Base Retraction. (A) Tongue base at rest prior to initiation of the pharyngeal swallow. (B) Complete approximation of the tongue base to the anteriorly displaced posterior pharyngeal wall.

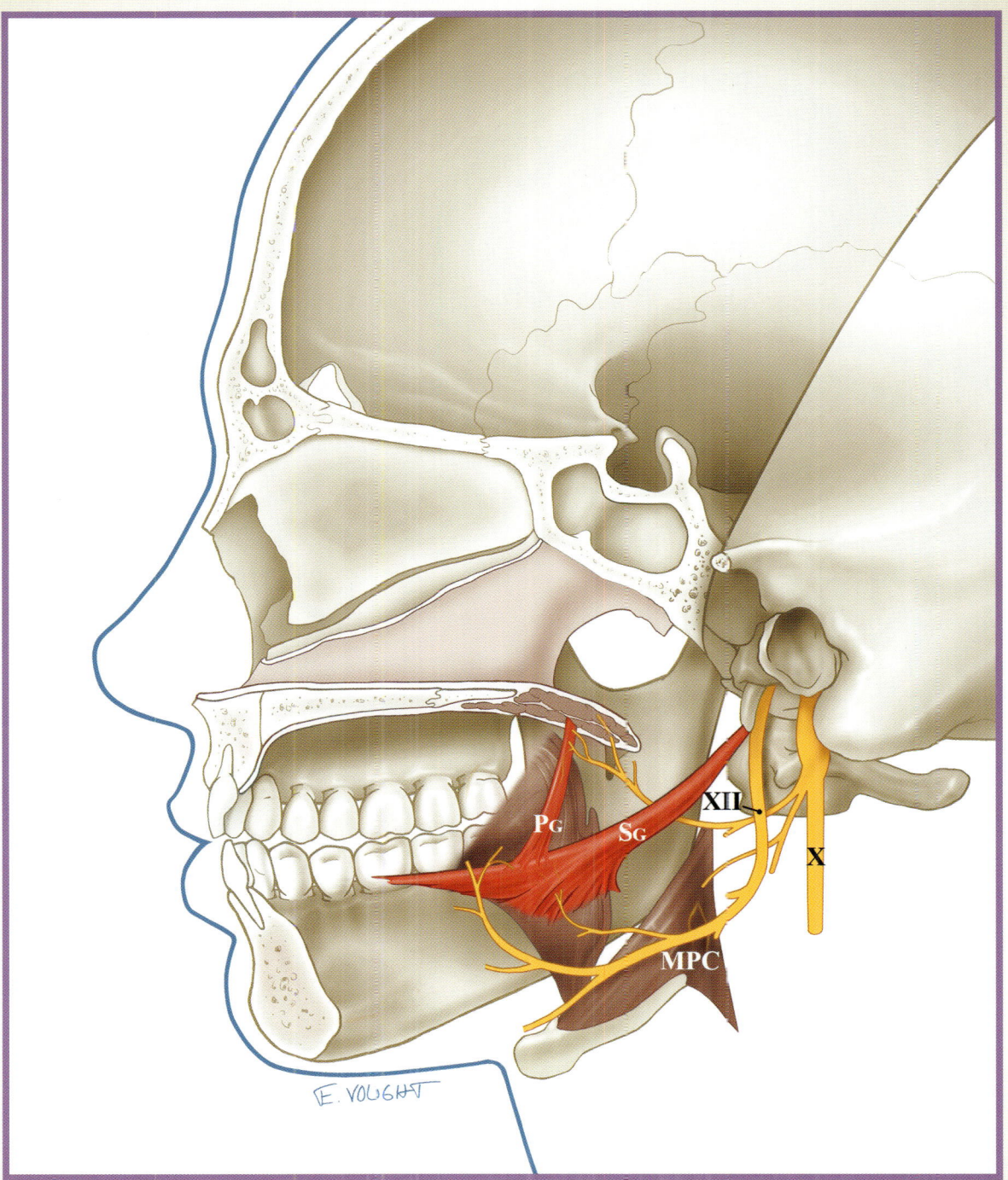

Figure 30 Muscles and innervation of Component 15 – Tongue Base Retraction. MPC-Middle pharyngeal constrictor; PG-Palatoglossus; SG-Styloglossus. X and XII refer to vagus and hypoglossus nerves, respectively.

Pharyngeal Domain
Component 16 – Pharyngeal Residue

Like oral residue (Component 5), pharyngeal residue represents a radiographic sign of a physiologic impairment that is significantly associated with the other components of pharyngeal impairment and several patient outcome measures. Despite the limitations of attempting to make 3-D cavity observations from a 2-D view, we were able to develop a visual perceptual metric that demonstrated good reliability and external validity. Pharyngeal residue is represented by any retention of contrast material on or within the pharyngeal structures that goes beyond lining or coating of structures. Rarely does residue isolate to a single location because patients typically do not have only one impaired component of swallowing function. Rather, most patients present with clusters of impairment that affect clearance of the bolus through the pharynx. Common locations for retention of contrast material in the pharynx include the valleculae (resulting from decreased tongue base retraction +/- impaired stripping action of the pharyngeal wall or impaired epiglottic inversion), posterior pharyngeal wall (resulting from impaired stripping wave +/- reduced PESO), and pyriform sinuses (resulting from impaired PESO distention, duration, or both).

Table 16 Muscles associated with MBSImP Component 16 – Pharyngeal Residue

Functional Group	Name	Innervation	Action
Pharyngoesophageal segment	Cricopharyngeus	CN X	Tonically contracted at rest but relaxes during swallowing to facilitate bolus passage
Pharyngeal constrictor muscles	Inferior pharyngeal constrictor		Applies positive pressure generation to the bolus tail through sequential contractions superiorly to inferiorly
	Superior pharyngeal constrictor		
	Middle pharyngeal constrictor		Applies positive pressure generation to the bolus tail through sequential contractions superiorly to inferiorly
Muscles of the base of tongue	Hyoglossus	CN XII	Retracts the base of tongue
	Styloglossus		
	Palatoglossus	CN X	
Long pharyngeal muscles	Stylopharyngeus	CN IX	Shortens and widens the pharynx
	Salpingopharyngeus	CN X	Elevates the larynx*
	Palatopharyngeus		
Suprahyoid muscles	Geniohyoid	C1	Elevates and moves the hyoid anteriorly contributing to superior-anterior movement trajectory
	Mylohyoid	CN V	
	Digastricus	Anterior belly: CN V	
	Stylohyoid**	CN VII	
Infrahyoid muscle	Thyrohyoid	C1	Elevates the thyroid cartilage to the hyoid

*Elevation of larynx displaces epiglottis to horizontal position.
**Although the stylohyoid is not a primary contributor, it assists in hyoid elevation.

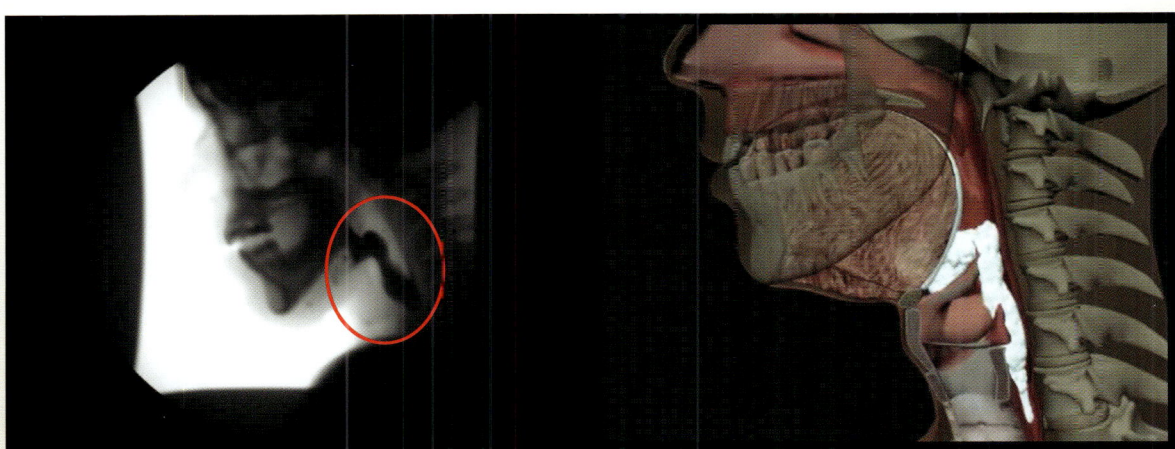

Figure 31 Videofluoroscopic and 3-D animated images demonstrating Component 16 – Pharyngeal Residue.

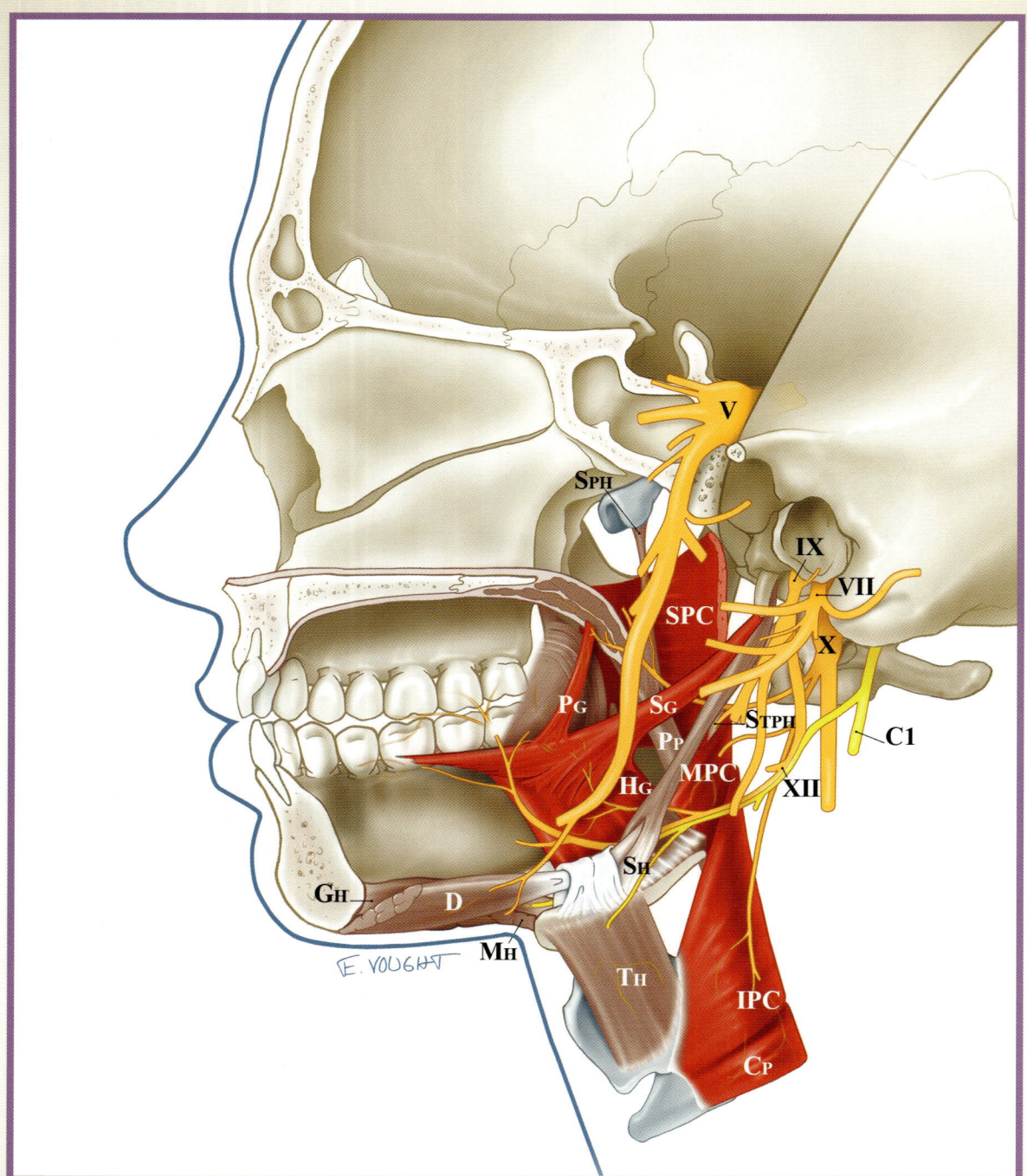

Figure 32 Muscles and innervation of Component 16 – Pharyngeal Residue. C$_P$-Cricopharyngeus; D-Digastricus (anterior belly); G$_H$-Geniohyoid; H$_G$-Hyoglossus; IPC-Inferior pharyngeal constrictor; MPC-Middle pharyngeal constrictor; M$_H$-Mylohyoid; P$_G$-Palatoglossus; P$_P$-Palatopharyngeus; S$_{PH}$-Salpingopharyngeus; S$_G$-Styloglossus; S$_H$-Stylohyoid; S$_{TPH}$-Stylopharyngeus; SPC-Superior pharyngeal constrictor; T$_H$-Thyrohyoid. V, VII, IX, X, and XII refer to trigeminal, facial, glossopharyngeal, vagus, and hypoglossal nerves, respectively. C1 refers to cervical spinal nerve 1.

Esophageal Domain
Component 17 – Esophageal Clearance (Upright Position)

The role of the SLP in assessment of esophageal function should be limited to observation of bolus clearance in the upright or semi-upright position because impairment in clearance has been shown to affect oropharyngeal swallowing behavior and treatment planning. The MBSS or MBSImP approach is not designed to evaluate esophageal *motility* or structural abnormalities. Motility testing requires the assessment of swallowing unassisted by gravity. SLPs are interested in gravity-assisted swallows, and in reality, make use of gravity assistance in selecting effective compensatory swallowing postures and strategies. Further, the MBSS is not sensitive for testing gastroesophageal reflux. Suspicion of reflux disorders should be brought to the attention of the referring physician and appropriate testing should be discussed. Lastly, the diagnosis of soft tissue structural lesions is outside the scope of SLP practice. The radiologist and patient's referring physician should immediately address any concerns regarding interrupted bolus flow in the esophagus or retrograde flow of the bolus from the esophagus into the pharynx.

Esophageal clearance is accomplished by a primary peristaltic wave that applies positive pressure to the bolus tail throughout the esophagus, similar to what occurs in the oral and pharyngeal cavities. The peristaltic wave includes a contraction of striated muscles that transitions to smooth muscle in and around the region of the aortic arch of the thoracic esophagus. This transition zone has been intently studied in the gastroenterological literature, because it is a region of decreased pressure and is a common location for contrast materials (particularly viscous and semisolids) to hesitate and remain for several seconds. The lower esophageal segment (LES) is comprised of smooth muscle fibers and relaxes simultaneous with CPM relaxation. However, unlike the PES, the LES does not require biomechanical action to permit opening for bolus passage into the stomach. The LES is a major anatomic and functional element of the gastroesophageal junction and creates a barrier to gastroesophageal reflux assisted by the crural diaphragm and intra-abdominal pressure.

Table 17 Muscles associated with MBSImP Component 17 – Esophageal Clearance

Name	Innervation	Action
Longitudinal and circular muscles of the esophagus	CN X Myenteric plexus	Primary and secondary peristaltic contraction

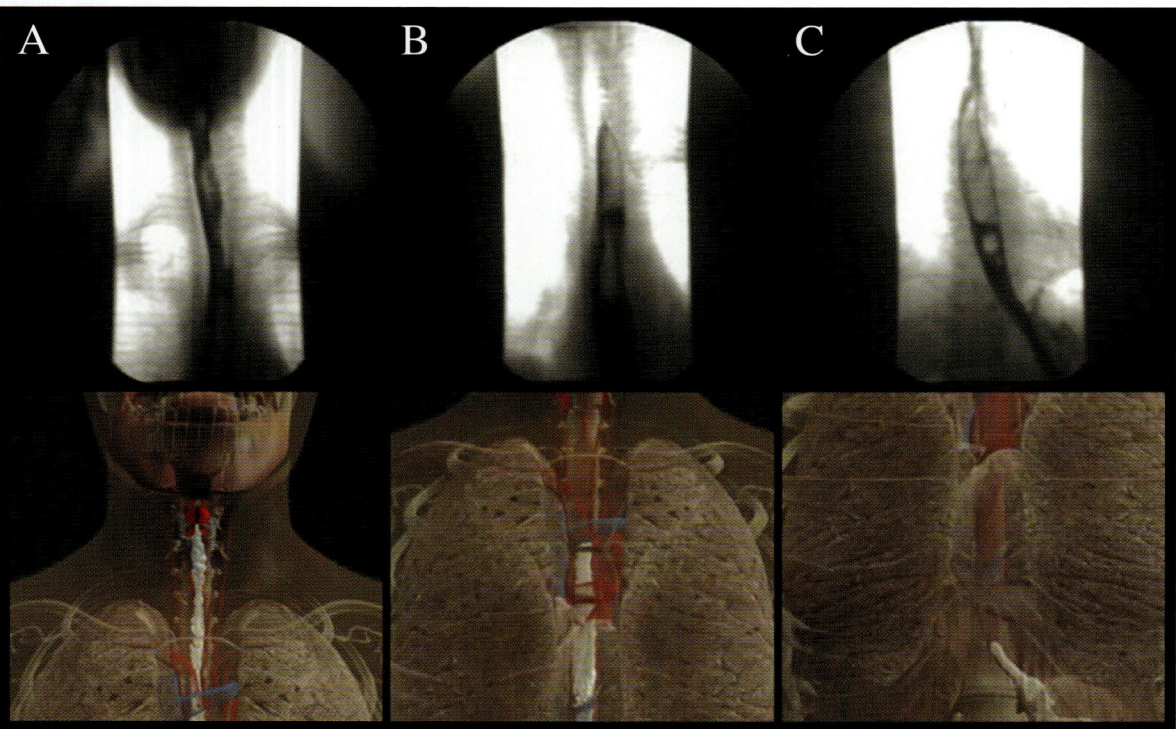

Figure 33 Videofluoroscopic and 3-D animated images demonstrating Component 17 – Esophageal Clearance-A/P View. (A) Bolus enters esophagus through PES. (B) Primary peristaltic wave applies positive pressure to the bolus tail throughout the esophagus. (C) Bolus enters stomach through LES.

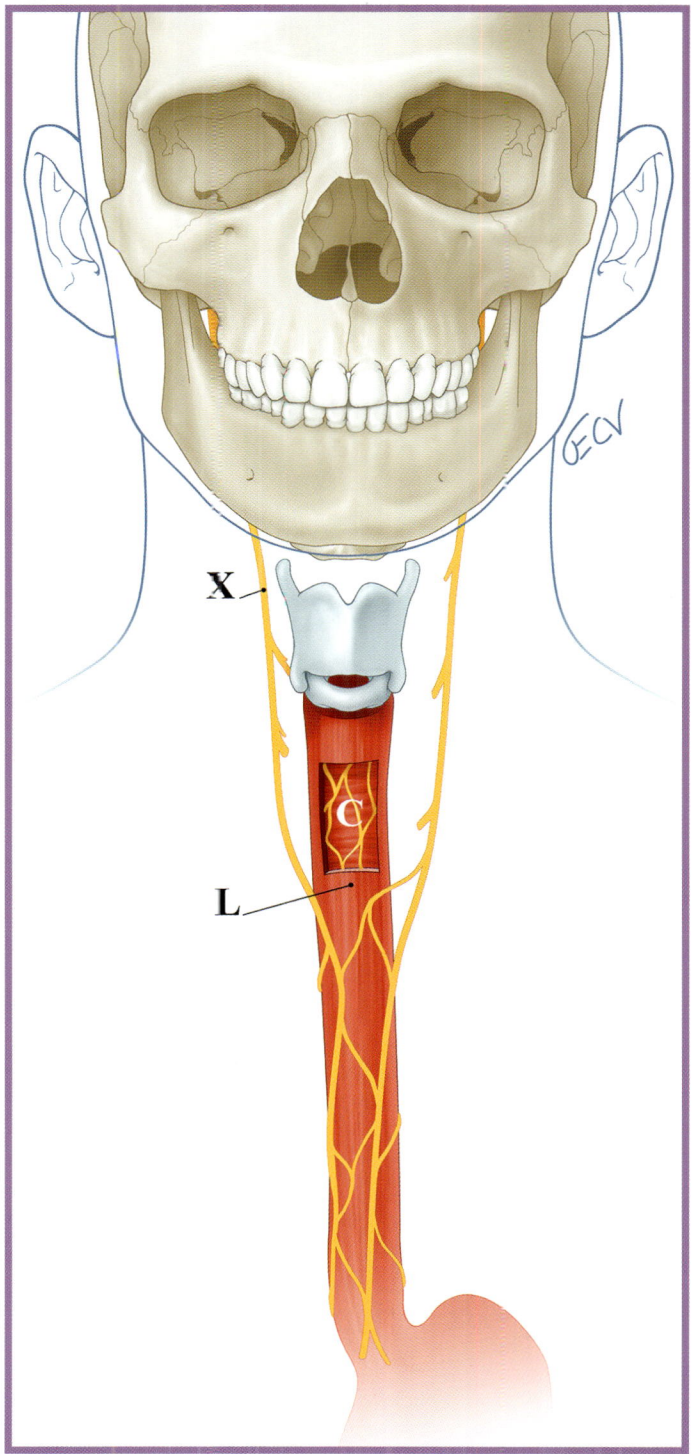

Figure 34 Muscles and innervation of Component 17 – Esophageal Clearance-A/P View. C-Circular muscles of esophagus; L-Longitudinal muscles of esophagus. X refers to vagus nerve.

Table 18 Cranial nerves critical to sensory innervation of the upper aerodigestive tract.

Cranial Nerve	Branch(es)	Receptive Field(s)	Swallowing Function
V (Trigeminal)	Maxillary (V2)	Palate Upper teeth and gums	Tactile Stereognosis } Bolus manipulation and preparation, and anterior oral containment
	Mandibular (V3)	Anterior tongue Lower teeth and gums	Tactile Stereognosis Proprioception } Bolus manipulation and preparation, and anterior oral containment Nociception Temperature
VII (Facial)	Chorda tympani	Anterior tongue Submandibular and sublingual glands	Taste Salivary production
IX (Glossopharyngeal)	Pharyngeal, lingual, and tonsillar	Glossopharyngeal (faucial) arches Back of tongue Parotid gland	Taste Tactile } Initiation of pharyngeal swallow and posterior oral containment Nociception Salivary production
X (Vagus)	Superior laryngeal nerve, internal branch	Base of tongue Valleculae Epiglottis Pharyngeal wall Aryepiglottic folds Ventricular folds Arytenoids True vocal folds Pyriform sinuses	Tactile → Initiation of pharyngeal swallow, and airway protection and clearance
	Recurrent laryngeal nerve	Subglottal larynx Trachea Bronchi	Tactile → Airway clearance

References and Suggested Readings

Allen JE, White C, Leonard R, Belafsky PC. Comparison of esophageal screen findings on videofluoroscopy with full esophagram results. *Head Neck.* 2012;34(2):264-269.

American Speech Language Hearing Association. Omnibus survey: Caseloads for speech-language pathologists. Rockville, MD: 2000.

Anapol F. Morphological and videofluorographic study of the hyoid apparatus and its function in the rabbit (Oryctolagus cuniculus). *J Morpho.* 1988;195:141-157.

Bisch, EM, Logemann JA, Rademaker AW, Kahrilas PJ, Lazarus CL. Pharyngeal effects of bolus volume, viscosity, and temperature in patients with dysphagia resulting from neurologic impairment and in normal subjects. *J Speech Lang Hear Res.* 1994;37(5):1041-1049.

Bonilha HS, Humphries K, Blair J, Hill EG, McGrattan K, Carnes BN, Huda W, Martin-Harris B. Radiation exposure time during MBSS: Influence of swallowing impairment severity, medical diagnosis, clinician experience, and standardized protocol use. *Dysphagia.* 2013;28(1):77-85.

Bonilha H, Blair J, Carnes B, Huda W, Humphries K, McGrattan K, Michel Y, Martin-Harris B. Preliminary investigation of the effect of pulse rate on judgments of swallowing impairment and treatment recommendations. *Dysphagia.* 2013;28(4):528-538.

Butler SG, Stuart A, Castell D, Russell GB, Koch K, Kemp S. Effects of age, gender, bolus condition, viscosity, and volume on pharyngeal and upper esophageal sphincter pressure and temporal measurements during swallowing. *J Speech Lang Hear Res.* 2009;52(1):240-253.

Brühlmann W. Impairments of swallowing: Diagnosis by cineradiography. *Diseases Abdomen Pelvis.* 2006;Part 1:40-44.

Castell DO. Manometric evaluation of the pharynx. *Dysphagia.* 1993;8(4):337-338.

Castell JA, Dalton CB, Castell DO. Pharyngeal and upper esophageal sphincter manometry in humans. *Am J Physiol.* 1990;258(2 Pt 1):G173-G178.

Castell JA, Castell DO. Modern solid state computerized manometry of the pharyngoesophageal segment. *Dysphagia.* 1993;8(3):270-275.

Cerenko D, McConnel FM, Jackson RT. Quantitative assessment of pharyngeal bolus driving forces. *Otolaryngol Head Neck Surg.* 1989;100(1):57-63.

Chi-Fishman G, Sonies B. Effects of systematic bolus viscosity and volume changes on hyoid movement kinematics. *Dysphagia.* 2002;17(4):278-287.

Cook IJ. Investigative techniques in the assessment of oral-pharyngeal dysphagia. *Dig Dis.* 1998;16(3):125-133.

Cook IJ, Dodds WJ, Dantas RO, et al. Timing of videofluoroscopic, manometric events, and bolus transit during the oral and pharyngeal phases of swallowing. *Dysphagia.* 1989;4:8-15.

Daggett A, Logemann J, Rademaker A, Pauloski B. Laryngeal penetration during deglutition in normal subjects of various ages. *Dysphagia.* 2006;21(4):270-274.

Daniels SK, Schroeder MF, DeGeorge PC, Corey DM, Rosenbek JC. Effects of verbal cue on bolus flow during swallowing. *Am J Speech Lang Pathol.* 2007;16(2):140-147.

DePippo KL, Holas MA, Reding MJ, Mandel FS, Lesser ML. Dysphagia therapy following stroke: A controlled trial *Neurology.* 1994;4499):1655-1660.

Dodds WJ, Man KM, Cook IJ, Kahrilas PJ, Stewart ET, Kern MK. Influence of bolus volume on swallow-induced hyoid movement in normal subjects. *Am J Roentgenol.* 1988;150:1307-1309.

Dodds WJ, Taylor AJ, Stewart ET, Kern MK, Logemann JA, Cook IJ. Tipper and dipper types of oral swallows. A*m J Roentgenol.* 1989;153(6):1197-1199.

Dodds WJ, Logemann JA, Stewart ET. Physiology and radiology of normal oral and pharyngeal phases of swallowing. *Am J Roentgenol.* 1990;154:953-963.

Dodds WJ, Stewart ET, Logemann JA. Radiologic assessment of abnormal oral and pharyngeal phases of swallowing. *Am J Roentgenol.* 1990;154:965-974.

Eisbruch A, Lyden T, Bradford CR, Dawson LA, Haxer MJ, Miller AE, Teknos TN, Chepeha DB, Hogiklyan ND, Terrell JE, Wolf GT. Objective assessment of swallowing dysfunction and aspiration after radiation concurrent with chemotherapy for head-and-neck cancer. *Int J Rad Oncol Biol Phys.* 2002;53(1):23-28.

Eisenhuber E, Schima W, Schober E, Pokieser P, Stadler A, Scharitzer M, Oschatz E. Videofluoroscopic assessment of patients with dysphagia: Pharyngeal retention is a predictive factor for aspiration. *Am J Roentgen.* 2002;178(2):393-398.

Ekberg O, Sijurjónsson SV. Movement of epiglottis during deglutition. A cineradiographic study. *Gastrointest Radiol.* 1982;7(2):101-107.

Ekberg O, Nylander G. Cineradiography in 45 patients with acute dysphagia. *Abdom Imaging.* 1983;8(1):295-302.

Ekberg O, Nylander G. Double-contrast examination of the pharynx. A*bdom Imaging.* 1985;10(1):263-271.

Ekberg O, Nylander G, Fork F-T, Sjöberg S, Birch-Iensen M, Hillarp B. Interobserver variability in cineradiographic assessment of pharyngeal function during swallow. *Dysphagia.* 1988;3(1):46-48.

Fattori B, Grosso M, Bongioanni P, Nacci A, Cristofani R, AlSharif A, Licitra R, Matteucci F, Rossi B, Rubello D. Assessment of swallowing by oropharyngeal scintigraphy in patients with amyotrophic lateral sclerosis. *Dysphagia.* 2006;21(4):280-286.

Focht, K.L. (2014). Variations in oropharyngeal swallowing physiology and aspiration risk in aging adults (dissertation). Medical University of South Carolina, Charleston, SC.

Frowen JJ, Cotton SM, Perry AR. The stability, reliability, and validity of videofluoroscopy measures for patients with head and neck cancer. *Dysphagia.* 2008;23(4):348-363.

Galli J, Valenza V, D'Alatri L, Reale F, Gajate AS, Di Girolamo S, Paludetti G. Postoperative dysphagia versus neurogenic dysphagia: Scintigraphic assessment. *Ann Otol Rhinol Laryngol.* 2003;112(1):20-28.

Green JR, Wang YT. Tongue-surface movement patterns during speech and swallowing. *J Acoust Soc Am.* 2003;113(5):2820-2833.

Groher ME, Crary MA, Carnaby (Mann) G, Vickers Z, Aguilar C. The impact of rheologically controlled materials on the identification of airway compromise on the clinical and videofluoroscopic swallowing examinations. *Dysphagia.* 2006;21(4):218-225.

Gullung J, Hill EG, Castell DO, Martin-Harris B. Oropharyngeal and esophageal swallowing impairment: Association and predictive value of Modified Barium Swallow Impairment Profile™ and combined multichannel intraluminal impedance-esophageal manometry. *Ann Oto Rhinol Laryngol.* 2012;121(11):738-745.

Gumbley F, Huckabee ML, Doeltgen SH, Witte U, Moran C. Effects of bolus volume on pharyngeal contact pressure during normal swallowing. *Dysphagia.* 2008;22(3):280-285.

Halpert RD, Feczko PJ, Spickler EM, Ackerman LV. Radiological assessment of dysphagia with endoscopic correlation. *Radiol.* 1985;157:599-602.

Hannam AG, Stavness I, Lloyd JE, Fels S. A dynamic model of jaw and hyoid biomechanics during chewing. *J Biomech.* 2008;41:1069-1076.

Hind JA, Nicosia MA, Roecker EB, Carnes ML, Robbins JA. Comparison of effortful and noneffortful swallows in healthy middle aged and older adults. *Arch Phys Med Rehabil.* 2001;82(12):1661-1665.

Hind JA, Gensler G, Brandt DK, Miller Gardner PJ, et al. Comparison of trained clinician ratings with expert ratings of aspiration on videofluoroscopic images from a randomized clinical trial. *Dysphagia*. 2009;24(2):211-217.

Huda W. What ER radiologists need to know about radiation risks. *Emergency Radiology*. 2009;16(5):335-341.

Jacob P, Kahrilas PJ, Logemann JA, Shav V, Ha T. Upper esophageal sphincter opening and modulation during swallowing. *Gastroenterol*. 1989;97(6):1469-1478.

Johnsson F, Shaw D, Gabb M, Dent J, Cook I. Influence of gravity and body position on normal oropharyngeal swallowing. *Am J Phys*. 1995;269(5 Pt 1):G653-G658.

Kaatzke-McDonald MN, Post E, Davis PJ. The effects of cold, touch, and chemical stimulation of the anterior faucial pillar on human swallowing. *Dysphagia*. 1996;11(3):198-206.

Kahrilas PJ, Logemann JA, Lin S, Ergun GA. Pharyngeal clearance during swallowing: A combined manometric and videofluoroscopic study. *Gastroenterology*. 1992;103(1):128-136.

Kahrilas PJ, Lin S, Logemann JA, Ergun GA, Facchini F. Deglutitive tongue action: Volume accommodation and bolus propulsion. *Gastroenterology*. 1993;104(1):152-162.

Kahrilas PJ, Lin, Rademaker AW, Logemann JA. Impaired deglutitive airway protection: A videofluoroscopic analysis of severity and mechanism. *Gastroenterology*. 1997;113(5):1457-1464.

Kelly AM, Drinnan MJ, Leslie P. Assessing penetration and aspiration: how do videofluoroscopy and fiberoptic endoscopic evaluation of swallowing compare? *Laryngoscope*. 2007;117(10):1723-1727.

Kendall KA, McKenzie S, Leonard RJ, Goncalves MI, Walker A. Timing of events in normal swallowing: A videofluoroscopic study. *Dysphagia*. 2000;15:74-83.

Kendall KA, Leonard RJ, McKenzie SW. Sequence variability during hypopharyngeal bolus transit. *Dysphagia*. 2003;18(2):85-91.

Kim Y, McCullough GH, Asp CW. Temporal measurements of pharyngeal swallowing in normal populations. *Dysphagia*. 2005;20(4):290-296.

Kim Y, McCullough GH. Maximum displacement in normal swallowing. *Dysphagia*. 2008;23(3):274-279.

Lazarus C, Logeman JA, Pauloski BR, et al. Effects of radiotherapy with or without chemotherapy on tongue strength and swallowing in patients with oral cancer. *Head Neck*. 2007;29(7) 632-637.

Leonard R, Kendall KA, McKenzie S. Structural displacements affecting pharyngeal constriction in nondysphagic elderly and nonelderly adults. *Dysphagia*. 2004;19(2):133-141.

Loeb M, McGreer A, McArthur M, et al. Risk factors for pneumonia and other lower respiratory tract infections in elderly residents of long-term care facilities. *Arch Intern Med*. 1999;159:2058-2064.

Logemann JA, Kahrilas PJ, Cheng J, Pauloski BR, Gibbons PJ, Rademaker AW, Lin S. Closure mechanisms of laryngeal vestibule during swallow. *Am J Physiol*. 1992;262(2 Pt 1):G338-G344.

Logemann JA, Pauloski BR, Rademaker AW, Colangelo LA, Kahrilas PJ, Smith CH. Temporal and biomechanical characteristics of oropharyngeal swallow in younger and older men. *J Speech Lang Hear Res*. 2000;43(5):1264-1274.

Logemann JA, Pauloski BR, Rademaker AW, Kahrilas PJ. Oropharyngeal swallow in younger and older women: Videofluoroscopic analysis. *J Speech Lang Hear Res*. 2002;45:434-445.

Logemann JA, Williams RB, Rademaker A, Pauloski BR, Lazarus C, Cook I. The relationship between observations and measures of oral and pharyngeal residue from videofluorography and scintigraphy. *Dysphagia*. 2005;20:226-231.

Marik PE, Kaplan D. Aspiration pneumonia and dysphagia in the elderly. *Chest*. 2003;124:328-336.

Martin BJW. *The influence of deglutition on respiration*. Unpublished doctoral dissertation. Northwestern University, Evanston, IL;1991.

Martin BJW, Logemann JA, Shaker R, Dodds W. Normal laryngeal valving patterns during three breath hold maneuvers: A pilot investigation. *Dysphagia*. 1993;8(1):11-20.

Martin BJ, Corlew MM, Wood H, et al. The association of swallowing dysfunction and aspiration pneumonia. *Dysphagia*. 1994;9:1-6.

Martin-Harris B. Do we have valid and reliable means of quantifying severity of oropharyngeal dysphagia? Moving toward standardization. *Persp Swallow Swallow Dis (Dysphagia)*. 2007;16(1):20-24.

Martin-Harris B, McMahon S, Haynes R. Aspiration and dysphagia: Pathophysiology and outcome. *Phonoscope*. 1998;2:125-132.

Martin-Harris B, Logemann J, McMahon S, Schleicher MA, Sandidge J. Clinical utility of the modified barium swallow. *Dysphagia*. 2000;15(3):136-141.

Martin-Harris B, Brodsky MB, Price CC, Michel Y, Walters B. Temporal coordination of laryngeal dynamics and breathing during swallowing: Single liquid swallows. *J Appl Physiol*. 2003;94:1735-1743.

Martin-Harris B, Michel Y, Castell D. Physiologic model of oropharyngeal swallowing revisited. *Otolaryngol Head Neck Surg*. 2005;133:234-240.

Martin-Harris B, Brodsky MB, Michel Y, Ford CL, Walters B, Heffner J. Breathing and swallowing dynamics across the adult lifespan. *Arch Otolaryngol Head Neck Surg*. 2005;131:762-770.

Martin-Harris B, Brodsky MB, Michel Y, Lee F-S, Walters B. Delayed initiation of the pharyngeal swallow: Normal variability in adult swallows. *J Speech Lang Hear Res*. 2007;50(3):585-594.

Martin-Harris B, Brodsky M, Michel Y, Castell D, Schleicher M, Sandidge J, Maxwell R, Blair J. MBS measurement tool of swallow impairment – MBSImP: Establishing a standard. *Dysphagia*. 2008;23(4):392-405.

Martin-Harris B, Jones B. The videofluorographic swallowing study. *Phys Med Rehabil Clin N Am*. 2008;19(4):769-785.

Massey BT. The use of intraluminal manometry to assess upper esophageal sphincter function. *Dysphagia*. 1993;8(4):339-344.

Matthew OP, Abu-Osba YK, Thach BT. Genioglossus muscle responses to upper airway pressure changes: Afferent pathways. *J Appl Physiol*. 1982;52(2):445-450.

McConnel FMS, Cerenko D, Hersch T, Weil LJ. Evaluation of pharyngeal dysphagia with manofluorography. *Dysphagia*. 1988;2(4):187-195.

McConnel FM, Guffin TN Jr, Cerenko D, KO AS. The effects of bolus flow on vertical pharyngeal pressure measurement in the pharyngoesophageal segment: Clinical significance. *Otolaryngol Head Neck Surg*. 1992;106(2):169-174.

McConnel FMS, Cerenko D, Mendelsohn MS. Manuflourographic analysis of swallowing. *Otolaryngol Clin N Am*. 1988;21:625-637.

McCullough GH, Wertz RT, Rosenbek JC, Mills RH, Ross KB, Ashford JR. Inter- and intrajudge reliability of a clinical examination of swallowing in adults. *Dysphagia*. 2000;15(2):58-67.

McLean D, Richard S, Collins L, Varas J. Thyroid dose measurements for staff involved in modified barium swallow exams. *Health Phys*. 2006;90(1):38-41.

Mettler FA, Bhargavan, M, Thomasden BR, Gilley DB, Lipoti JA, et al. Nuclear medicine exposure in the United States, 2005-2007: Preliminary results. *Sem Nuclear Med*. 2008;38(5):384-391.

Mettler FA, Bhargavan, M, Faulkner K, Gilley DB, Gray JE, et al. Radiologic and nuclear medicine studies in the United States and worldwide: Frequency, radiation dose, and comparison with other radiation sources-1950-2007. *Radiology*. 2009;253:520-531.

Miller LS, Dai Q, Sweitzer BA, Thangada V, Kim JK, Thomas B, Parkman H, Soliman AM. Evaluation of the upper esophageal sphincter (UES) using simultaneous high-resolution endoluminal sonography (HRES) and manometry. *Dig Diseases Sci.* 2004;49(5):703-709.

Molfenter SM, Steele CM. Physiological variability in the deglutition literature: Hyoid and laryngeal kinematics. *Dysphagia.* 2011;26(1):67-74.

Moro L, Cazzani C. Dynamic swallowing study and radiation dose to patients. *La Radiologia Medica.* 2006;111(1):123-129.

National Council on Radiation Protection & Measurements. Report No. 100-Exposure of the U.S. population from diagnostic medical radiation. Bethesda, MD;1988.

O'Donoghue S, Bagnall A. Videofluoroscopic evaluation in the assessment of swallowing disorders in paediatric and adult populations. *Folia Phoniatr Logogop.* 1999;51:158-171.

Olsson R, Nilsson H, Ekberg O. Simultaneous videoradiography and computerized pharyngeal manometry-videomanometry. *Acta Radiologica.* 1994;35(1):30-34.

Olsson R, Castell JA, Castell DO, Ekberg O. Solid-state computerized manometry improves diagnostic yield in pharyngeal dysphagia: Simultaneous videoradiography and manometry in dysphagia patients with normal barium swallows. *Abnormal Imaging.* 1995;20(3):230-235.

Pearson WG, Hindson DF, Langmore SE, Zumwalt AC. Evaluating swallowing muscles essential for hyolaryngeal elevation by using muscle functional magnetic resonance imaging. *IJROBP.* 2013;85:735-740.

Pearson WG, Langmore SE, Zumwalt AC. Evaluating the structural properties of suprahyoid muscles and their potential for moving the hyoid. *Dysphagia.* 2011;26(4):345-351.

Pearson WG, Langmore SE, Yu LB, Zumwalt AC. Structural analysis of muscles elevating the hyolaryngeal complex. *Dysphagia.* 2012;27(4):445-451.

Périé S, Laccourreye L, Flahault A, Hazebroucq V, Chaussade S, St. Guily JL. Role of videoendoscopy in assessment of pharyngeal dysfunction in oropharyngeal dysphagia: Comparison with videofluoroscopy and manometry. *Laryngoscope.* 1998;108(11):1712-1716.

Perlman AL, Schultz JG, VanDaele DJ. Effects of age, gender, bolus volume, and bolus viscosity on oropharyngeal pressure during swallowing. *J Appl Phsyiol.* 1993;75:33-37.

Perlman AL, Palmer PM, McCulloch TM, Van Daele DJ. Electromyographic activity from human laryngeal, pharyngeal, and submental muscles during swallowing. *J Appl Phys.* 1999;86(5):1663-1669.

Perlman AL, VanDaele DJ, Otterbacher MS. Quantitative assessment of hyoid bone displacement from video images during swallowing. *J Speech Lang Hear Res.* 1995;38(3):579-585.

Pouderoux P, Kahrilas PJ. Deglutitive tongue force modulation by volition, volume, and viscocity in humans. *Gastroenterol.* 1995;108(5):1418-1426.

Rademaker AW, Pauloski BR, Colangelo LA, Logemann JA. Age and volume effects on liquid swallowing function in normal women. *J Speech Lang Hear Res.* 1998;41:275-284.

Reddy NP, Canilang EP, Grotz RC, Rane MB, Casterline J, Costarella BR. Biomechanical quantification for assessment and diagnosis of dysphagia. *IEEE Eng Med Biol Mag.* 1988;7(3):16-20.

Robbins J, Coyle J, Rosenbek J, Roecker E, Wood, J. Differentiation of normal and abnormal airway protection during swallowing using the penetration-aspiration scale. *Dysphagia.* 1999;14(4):228-232.

Robbins J, Hamilton JW, Lof GL, Kempster GB. Oropharyngeal swallowing in normal adults of different ages. *Gastroenterol.* 1992;103:823-829.

Rosenbek JC, Robbins J, Roecker EV, Coyle JL, Woods JL. A penetration-aspiration scale. *Dysphagia.*1996;11:93-98.

Sia I, Carvajal P, Carnaby-Mann GD, Crary MA. Measurement of hyoid and laryngeal displacement in video fluoroscopic swallowing studies: variability, reliability, and measurement error. *Dysphagia.* 2012;27(2):192-197.

Singh V, Berry S, Brockbank MJ, Frost RA, Tyler SE, Owens D. Investigation of aspiration: Milk nasendoscopy versus videofluoroscopy. *European Arch Oto-Rhino-Laryngol.* 2009;266(4):543-545.

Staff DM, Shaker R. Videoendoscopic evaluation of supraesophageal dysphagia. *Curr Gastroenterol Rep.* 2001;3(3):200-205.

Stroudley J, Walsh M. Radiological assessment of dysphagia in Parkinson's disease. *British J Radiol.* 1991;64:890-893.

Wheeler, KM, Chiara T, Sapienza CM. Surface electromyographic activity of the submental muscles during swallow and expiratory pressure threshold training tasks. *Dysphagia.* 2007;22:108-116.

Wilson RD, Howe EC. A cost-effectiveness analysis of screening methods for dysphagia after stroke. *Phys Med Rehabil.* 2012;4:273-282.

Vandaele DJ, Perlman AL, Cassell MD. Intrinsic fibre architecture and attachments of the human epiglottis and their contributions to the mechanism of deglutition. *J Anat.* 1995;186:1-15.

Zhang S, Olthoff A, Frahm J. Real-time magnetic resonance imaging of normal swallowing. *JMRI.* 2012; 35:1372-9.

About the Author

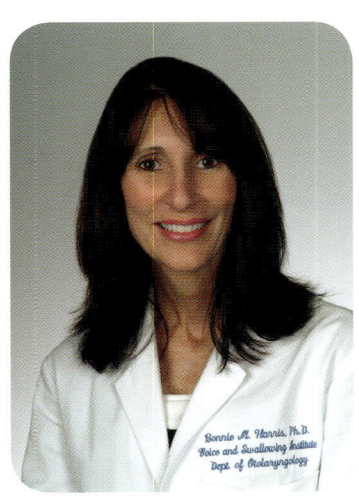

Bonnie Martin-Harris, Ph.D., CCC-SLP, BCS-S, ASHA Fellow

Dr. Martin-Harris is an internationally renowned lecturer, researcher, and clinician. At the Medical University of South Carolina (MUSC), she is Professor within the Department of Otolaryngology-Head and Neck Surgery, and Professor within the Department of Health and Rehabilitation Science. Additionally, she is Director of the Doctoral Program in Health and Rehabilitation Science, and Director of the MUSC Evelyn Trammell Institute for Voice and Swallowing. Dr. Martin-Harris is an ASHA Fellow. She is a Past-President of the Dysphagia Research Society and Past-Chair of the American Board of Swallowing and Swallowing Disorders (BCS-S).

Dr. Martin-Harris led a five-year investigation to test reliability, content, construct, and external validity of a new MBS study tool (MBSImP) to be used to quantify swallowing impairment. This research was the impetus for the MBSImP approach and was published in *Dysphagia* in 2008. She then led the development of the MBSImP standardized clinical online training that was released in 2011. Presently, Dr. Martin-Harris continues to conduct research on swallowing and swallowing disorders and presents internationally on the use of standardized and evidence-based practices in speech-language pathology.

For more information on the
MBSImP Standardized Clinical Online Training
please visit
www.NorthernSpeech.com/MBSImP

NOTES